Advance praise for
Encounters with the Invisible

"Dorothy Wall's riveting account of her experience of chronic fatigue syndrome (CFS) will provide companionship for those afflicted and serve as an eye-opener for those who are not."
—ANNE HUNSAKER HAWKINS, Director,
The Doctors Kienle Center for Humanistic Medicine at Penn State's College of Medicine, and author of *A Small Good Thing: Stories of Children with HIV and Those Who Care for Them*

"Wall is a tour guide, leading us through the mysterious grottos of illness. Seamless prose carries the reader along the twists and turns of the body's mutiny. This book is for doctors, patients, and indeed all readers."
—DANIELLE OFRI, M.D., Editor-in-Chief
of the *Bellevue Literary Review*, and author of *Incidental Findings: Lessons from My Patients in the Art of Medicine*

"Wall's intimate disclosures, wise observations, and eloquent style shed light on an astonishing variety of topics—cultural, historical, anthropological, personal—and deliver a satisfying intellectual and emotional experience. The hopeful conclusion celebrates Ms. Wall's achievement—in writing the book and recovering sufficiently to embrace the simplest of life's pleasures."
—K. KIMBERLY McCLEARY, President & CEO,
CFIDS Association of America

Encounters
with the Invisible

MEDICAL HUMANITIES
Thomas Mayo, series editor

ENCOUNTERS
with the
INVISIBLE

Unseen Illness, Controversy,
and Chronic Fatigue Syndrome

DOROTHY WALL

*Afterword
by Nancy Klimas, M.D.*

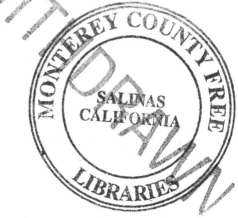

Southern Methodist University Press
Dallas

Requests for permission to reproduce material from this work should be sent to:
Rights and Permissions
Southern Methodist University Press
PO Box 750415
Dallas, Texas 75275-0415

Grateful acknowledgment is made to the following publications in which chapters of this
book, in altered form, first appeared: *Bellevue Literary Review, Sonora Review, Nimrod:
International Journal, Clackamas Literary Review, Under the Sun, Flyway: A Literary Review,
Puerto del Sol, San Francisco Chronicle Magazine,* and
Stricken: Voices from the Hidden Epidemic of Chronic Fatigue Syndrome,
edited by Peggy Munson (New York: The Haworth Press, 2000).

Cover photograph: "Hartwig House, Truro, 1976" by Joel Meyerowitz
Cover and text design by Kellye Sanford

Library of Congress Cataloging-in-Publication Data

Wall, Dorothy, 1948-
    Encounters with the invisible : unseen illness, controversy, and chronic fatigue syndrome /
Dorothy Wall ; afterword by Nancy Klimas.
    p. cm. — (Medical humanities)
    Includes index.
    ISBN 0-87074-504-2 (alk. paper)
    1. Wall, Dorothy, 1948—Health. 2. Chronic fatigue syndrome—Patients—California—
Biography. I. Title. II. Series.

RB150.F37W35 2005
362.196'0478'0092—dc22
[B]

                                                                                    2005051665

Printed in the United States of America on acid-free paper
10   9   8   7   6   5   4   3   2   1

For Bill and Lisa,
and for all those who live with and despite CFIDS

Acknowledgments

To write a book while ill is in some ways a reckless venture, requiring an exceptional level of support and commitment from others. First and foremost among my pillars has been my partner, Bill Barnes, without whose steady and extraordinary help this book would still be languishing in files and folders and a handful of literary magazines. As a political scientist, he saw when I first handed him a few fledgling pages the importance of engaging the medical and cultural issues behind CFIDS, and piled my bed with books he thought I should read and articles he pulled from the Web. He did an enormous amount of research for me over many years, traipsing to numerous libraries and searching the Internet for articles, saving me from having to use the computer for anything other than the actual writing. He edited each chapter multiple times, bringing clarity and insight to my sometimes muddy prose. He encouraged me when I doubted, brought meals to my bedside when I was exhausted, ran to the post office or photocopy shop whenever needed, and gave sustenance in countless ways. Bill is the dream of every writer, a partner who challenges me intellectually and supports me emotionally and logistically, available day and night. I can never thank him enough.

The book began as fragments and terse essays that I handed, unsolicited, to visiting friends. Their feedback and encouragement meant a great deal: Susan Hoffman, Nancy Bardacke, and Sherrie Hansen read early drafts and were kind enough to tell me I should keep working. As the drafts began hinting at a book, other friends supplied camaraderie, insightful comments, hot and sour soup, and that essential food of writers, enthusiasm: Susan Page, Elizabeth Nelson, Judy Turiel, Patricia Walker, Kathy Eisman.

I will always be indebted to longtime friend Peggy Schaefer, who didn't live to see her book published, nor mine, but whose generous bequest allowed me time to write in the final year of work. She provided respite more than once, and in many ways, in the course of my illness; her graciousness meant more than she perhaps knew. A much appreciated grant from the Money for Women/Barbara Deming Memorial Fund, Inc., also gave the crucial gift of time to write.

My thanks to editor Caroline Pincus, who prodded, questioned, and offered smart feedback at that midway point when a book is like a half-completed sculpture. A huge, heartfelt thanks goes to Peggy Munson for all she did to help, even as she struggled with her own illness. She pushed my thinking, provided superb editing, assisted with research, and came up with needed information in a pinch. The book would not have taken shape the way it did without her fine editorial eye and broad knowledge of CFIDS.

I thank Dr. Anthony Komaroff, Dr. David Bell, Dr. Carol Jessop, and Dr. Leonard Jason for squeezing time from busy schedules to talk with me and answer my many questions. Their knowledge and perspective were invaluable. Roger Burns gave insight into the name-change controversy. Kim Kenney McCleary was especially forbearing, willing to give me a crash course in CFIDS research and advocacy, to endure endless questions, type e-mails when she was swamped with work, ferret out research materials, and dispense constant encouragement. I greatly appreciate her support for my book as well as her tireless advocacy work, so vital to everyone with CFIDS. Marcia Harmon and many others at the CFIDS Association took time to dig up information and mail materials. They, along with so many other advocates out there, are the practical angels of the CFIDS community, and I thank them all for their dedication.

I'm deeply grateful to my agent, Felicia Eth, the kind of ally every writer wants: shrewd in business, wise in counsel—and she answers the phone. She saw the potential in my early drafts when it took a leap of faith to do so, and remained committed despite commercial publishing trends. I've been nourished by her friendship and her consistent belief in my work.

I thank my editor at SMU Press, Kathryn Lang, who made me glad to have an expert in my corner. Her e-mails began and ended my day for many months, and I came to rely on her warmth, skill, and professionalism. Her agile editing made the book more polished and readable, and she made the editing experience a pleasure. I also thank at SMU Press George Ann Ratchford for her excellent help and patience in shepherding the book through the production and marketing phases, and Keith Gregory for all his behind-the-scenes efforts. Thanks to Dave Bullen, whose well-placed words enabled me to find the cover art while lying in bed, to Jean Hohl, who gave up a weekend to perform the mechanical magic of converting my disk to Word, and to Paul Spragens for his sharp copyediting.

My sisters—Suzanne Orcutt, Alice Williams, Martha Wall, and Laura Wall—have been a stalwart source of support, love, editing, fact-finding, disk storage, and loyalty throughout my illness and the writing of this book. I'm grateful to them all. Though my mother, Barbara Mortensen, died before I began the book, her spirit and creativity are threaded throughout.

Finally, I thank my daughter, Lisa Warsen, companion, helpmate, friend. She handled with aplomb the role reversal that a mother's illness brings, didn't flinch when I incorporated her notes and words into my story, and always cheered me on. She brightens my life every day. No mother could ask for more. Among her many gifts, she has brought into our lives a wonderfully spirited son-in-law, Dennis Warsen, and a sticky-fingered and exuberant grandson, Zane, who reminds us why we go through all we do.

Author's Note

E ncounters with the Invisible: Unseen Illness, Controversy, and Chronic Fatigue Syndrome chronicles the evolution of personal, public, and medical understanding of an illness, and in doing so it tracks the evolution of an illness name. In 1988, the CDC officially affixed the label chronic fatigue syndrome (CFS) to this illness, a trivializing name, reviled by patients, that has contributed to widespread misconceptions about the disease. Soon after, many patients and advocates adopted the name chronic fatigue and immune dysfunction syndrome (CFIDS) to call attention to the immune system component of the illness. Some, especially in Canada, Australia, and Western Europe, had already been using myalgic encephalomyelitis (ME), a term established in the medical literature since the 1950s. More recently, in 2003, a panel of experts issued a Canadian clinical case definition using the dual name ME/CFS, and many now use this composite. In this book I have used CFS and CFIDS, since these are the names I and others around me were using at the time I was writing. I recognize the power of language and the volatility of the name-change debate, and hope that my detailed exploration of the name-change movement in Chapters Four and Fourteen will illuminate the complex issues at stake.

Contents

Introduction

When a strange, flulike illness began its insidious spread through the United States in the late 1970s and early '80s, in the dark undertow of AIDS, few people noticed. In Charlotte, North Carolina; Key West, Florida; San Francisco, California; Lyndonville, New York; Boston, Massachusetts—across the country previously healthy people were showing up in medical offices complaining of profound fatigue, difficulty with memory and concentration, sore throats, swollen lymph glands, muscle aches and weakness, headaches, low-grade fevers. Puzzled physicians ordered lab tests that revealed little. They sent their patients home, assuring them they'd get better in a week or two.

But patients didn't get better. Clinician and researcher Anthony Komaroff of Harvard Medical School, who first saw patients with this illness at the Brigham and Women's Hospital in 1977, was astonished. "The fact that you could get a common virus and still be ill a year later—that was striking."[1] This mysterious epidemic didn't kill its victims, didn't offer an obvious lesion or low blood count, and didn't arouse much medical or epidemiological interest. Many doctors wagged their heads at their patients' "emotional" problems. When internists Paul Cheney and Daniel Peterson in Incline Village, Nevada, asked the Centers for Disease Control and Prevention (CDC) in Atlanta to investigate a cluster of some ninety patients in June of 1985, it took three months for investigators to arrive.[2] Yet victims of this illness were severely debilitated, often unable to work or even to walk several blocks.

It would be 1988 before the CDC finally named the confounding illness "chronic fatigue syndrome" (CFS). Even then CFS was subject to psychiatric explanations by physicians, disbelief by family, coworkers, and friends of those who were ill, and media ridicule as the "yuppie flu." It was overlaid with judgment and myth: shirker, blockage in the fourth chakra, unresolved childhood issues. This disastrous illness was a silent epidemic, kept invisible by lack of official acknowledgment and concern. Victims suffered with little recognition or support. And it was an epidemic that would grow—to over 800,000 adults in the United States by 1999, twice as many as have multiple sclerosis.

Susan Sontag has famously written of illness as "the night-side of life, a more onerous citizenship. Everyone who is born holds dual citizenship, in the kingdom of the well and in the kingdom of the sick."[3] Illness is indeed a country apart, one that most of us will someday visit. To be seriously ill is to inhabit a world radically different from that of the healthy. Illness is not one country, though, but many, each differently contoured. CFS and other controversial, perhaps overlapping, illnesses—fibromyalgia, Gulf War syndrome, multiple chemical sensitivity, candidiasis, chronic Lyme disease—exist in a country apart from cancer or measles, diseases recognized and treatable by the medical establishment. Those with contested illnesses reside in a lonely, disparaged country of their own.

Ironically, these marginalized illnesses may be the most consequential for today's medical practice, exposing the inadequacy of the reductive, pathology-oriented biomedical model. Dr. Arthur Kleinman, a Harvard psychiatrist and anthropologist who has written extensively about chronic illness, notes with wry understatement, "The care of chronic illness is not one of the great success stories of modern medicine."[4] While scientific medicine has vanquished an impressive roster of infectious diseases—diphtheria, rheumatic fever, polio, syphilis, TB, measles—in First World countries at least, we remain subject to an array of chronic illnesses that make biomedicine appear far less grand. While news stories tout the successes of molecular science, gene mapping, and high-tech interventions to treat disease, there's another, untold story within today's medical landscape. It is the story of the growing number of chronic, controversial illnesses poorly served by today's biomedical, mechanistic approach to disease.

As patients with these complex illnesses flood medical offices, modern medicine is witnessing a disastrous collision between patient needs and experiences, and physician orientation and practices. To have CFS is to be caught in this collision.

The day I was drawn into this social and medical drama was an innocuous one, as life-changing moments often are, their explosive significance revealed only in retrospect. My pivotal moment came amid a swirl of green paint on a June day in 1980. I had awakened that morning feeling sluggish, fluish. It was a fine early summer day and I was flush with ambition, having just completed my M.A. coursework in creative writing and quit my bookstore job. From my upstairs flat on Claremont Avenue in Oakland, despite my lethargy, I lugged a can of Kelly green paint and a jar of paint remover out to the driveway and set about stripping a small bookcase and painting a Fifties-style desk with tapered legs, a friend's castoff, for my daughter. At eight, she'd been dropping broad hints that she was overdue for an upgrade from her baby furniture.

Climbing roses, waxy white, bloomed along the fence. Cars whooshed by. I relished the day as one of homey chores and accomplishments, a day leaning toward a bright future. I had only to take my M.A. orals and was set to plunge into the itinerant college teaching circuit in the fall, a rather optimistic ambition that involved commuting all around the Bay Area, stitching a pastiche of part-time positions into a full-time job that paid less than cleaning motels. Nonetheless, visions of my students pouring out their poems overrode the skeptical stares of those fellow poets who had long since defected to write technical manuals. I was as sure that I could make a go of it as I was that I could paint that desk.

Sinking with fatigue, I sloshed a too bright green—what had I been thinking?—across the desk. With each glistening brushstroke I sank further, my head strangely fibrous, my body a wooden bulk I struggled to animate. Sunlight off the paint was blinding, the fumes peculiarly refracted, as if I could smell each distinct molecule. I kept working until the last green stroke melted into a plasticized sheen, then went in to lie down.

An exhaustion thick as sod settled in my head and limbs. I'd had mononucleosis at the end of 1978—a rocky time of divorce, grad school, work, single-parenting—and had never fully recovered. Completing my M.A. coursework had been a constant exercise in mustering my flagging strength. But this weariness had a new quality—detached, unanchored, yet rock-heavy—and a feeling of fogginess and confusion I'd never experienced.

By the time I dragged myself to the doctor some days later I had bronchitis and a sinus infection to boot. Even with antibiotics coursing through my blood, this illness defied anything I'd known. I remember waking one morning after a couple of weeks, feeling somewhat better, the sun glinting through bamboo shades. I made my oatmeal, dressed, and settled in a lit spot on the bed to immerse myself in Christina Rossetti's poems in preparation for my orals. I can do this, I thought. I began to lose myself in Rossetti's lurid Victorian fantasies and renunciatory laments, "I dwell alone—I dwell alone, alone."

One hour later I put the book down. My head was spinning. The words stopped taking shape, my vision cut by a white swath of confusion. I felt inside a fog bank, clarity and sharp outlines somewhere beyond, out of reach. I couldn't absorb another sentence. Rossetti landed upside down; my head landed on the pillow. I'd been able to function for one hour. I lay flat on my back the rest of the day.

I don't have any idea how I managed that summer—how I fed my daughter, got her to school, finished writing that uninspired creative writing workbook that was paying my summer bills. Did friends do my marketing? I don't remember. But I do recall the day in September when I woke and thought, with the relief that comes with a gush of spring air, I think I'm well. The next day I was hit again, as if by some invisible, inhabiting force. I was as ill as I'd been two months earlier, with the exact same symptoms. My doctor doubled my antibiotics. It did no good. I have an enduring picture of one doctor after another peering at me with that poker face that means they're madly trying to compute the subtext: Was I a malingerer? Did I evidence emotional imbalance? Was I having family problems?

And so it went for the next six years: a massive, recurring, viral-like illness, a strange, dogged malaise that left doctors shrugging, that shadowed my days even as I hauled my body onward, to teach—one hour in front of my class left my throat raw, my chest burning—to tuck my daughter in bed, even to party with friends. I was only thirty-two, otherwise healthy, and had things to do. I wasn't about to let a virus keep me from unreeling the myth of a self-made life. Over time the symptoms became somewhat less severe, the periods between flare-ups lengthened, but for all those years my viral cohort kept up its relentless cycle.

I entered illness blind, not knowing what line I had crossed or what lay ahead, no different than anyone poised at the beginning of a new endeavor—and despite the image it conjures of limp passivity, illness *is* an endeavor, an undertaking. I didn't know that I would never again reside wholly and without thought in the land of the well, that this nascent life of illness wasn't going to abate, that I had exchanged the energetic body of my childhood for one that lugged an iron weight on its back. I had yet to learn that for every attempt to override what smote me, for every determined, carry-on day, my body would exact its revenge, or that I would be one of many who were similarly ill, yet isolated and alone, the extent of my body's distress unknown even to myself.

In 1869 American neurologist George Beard characterized neurasthenia, a fatiguing illness suggestive of CFS, as the "Central Africa of medicine—an unexplored territory into which few men enter."[5] Leaving aside the smug taint of American chauvinism, Beard's description of this dark interior continent is evocative of the unmapped territory of CFS. Scientific medicine has shrunk the acreage of that obscure continent of unexplained illness; it has not abolished it. Those of us with CFS still inhabit this murky space.

More than two decades after CFS emerged, we still don't know its cause or pathophysiology, though there's a growing body of research, the scientific language of suffering, revealing abnormalities of the neurologic, immune, autonomic, and endocrine systems. Many researchers and clinicians now suspect that CFS—also called chronic fatigue and immune dysfunction syndrome (CFIDS) and myalgic encephalomyelitis (ME)—may be a cluster of illnesses with one or more pathogens, chemical and environmental exposures, stress and injury, and genetics all possibly playing a role. Says clinician Paul Cheney, "I believe that CFS is a heterogeneous illness that can be produced by a variety of triggers. But there was some *new* triggering agent in the 1970s."[6]

I've been astonished to learn that I'm part of a broad epidemiological map, not alone as I had thought for so many years. And fascinated to discover, too, stories of nineteenth- and twentieth-century epidemics—nineteenth-century neurasthenia, the L.A. County epidemic of 1934, London's Royal Free disease in 1954, among others—whose profiles are remarkably similar to CFIDS: clusters of previously healthy people struck with flulike symptoms followed by years of debilitation.

All of us in this current epidemic have company, in the present and the past.

By 1986–87, my recurring flulike symptoms—the massive brain fog, swollen glands, earaches, and sore throats—slowly began to lift, like evaporating dampness. I had days when I could step outside to see a sharp, crystalline world instead of an overwhelming, blurry cacophony, my head miraculously unclouded. I fell in love, occasionally walked as much as three miles, even traipsed along the canals of Venice with my new partner, Bill. I remember one day in 1989 saying to him with the sense of a sweeping, remarkable mountaintop vision as I looked back on the last nine years, "I'm still exhausted much of the time, but I don't get sick anymore." Some days I was merely tired. A few days a year I felt amazingly, blessedly normal.

Ah, the deceit of normalcy, the false hope of busyness. My frenetic professional life—teaching writing classes and workshops, speaking at conferences, coauthoring a book, consulting privately with writers—swept me along in its tow. By the early 1990s I was once again sick most of the year. I knew I was overextended. I kept promising myself I would rest "after I'm finished with . . . ." I didn't understand my body's growing complaints, the calamity building in every muscle and bone, didn't know I could become more ill than I'd been.

I was face-to-face with CFIDS's disturbing profile: it is often circular as much as linear, characterized by alternating cycles of improvement and relapse. Dr. Paul Cheney describes a three-phase model of CFIDS which is useful to understand its overall pattern.[7] The onset or trigger phase is characterized by acute, flulike symptoms that leave patients reeling, often bedridden, with what they describe as the most massive flu they've ever had. Within several months or several years, instead of resolving, the illness evolves into classic CFIDS, or the triad phase, so called because of its triad of symptoms: the patient may be somewhat improved, but still suffers overwhelming fatigue, a brain that doesn't work, and a body that hurts all over. Five or ten years later the patient enters phase three, the dynamic injury phase, in which brain function is improved, pain has subsided to a lower level, but damage to multiple body systems continues to limit mental and physical activity. While patients feel less sick overall, they don't return to the levels of work or exercise they maintained before becoming ill.

These three phases exist along a continuum and often overlap. Even in phase three patients may have swollen glands and a sore throat for weeks, even months. Their muscle and joint pain may still flare up. But the predominant feature is that they can't engage in a normal level of activity, and if they exceed their limits, they'll relapse. Some people experience a gradual rather than acute onset, making these phases more fuzzy, but the person can usually identify, in hindsight at least, a similar overall pattern.

If the fall into illness, the destruction of the ordinary, is capricious and sudden, the rebuilding of a life is deliberate and painstaking. This book focuses primarily on my rude confrontation with acute illness beginning in the fall of 1995, when I became more ill than ever, and the slow restitching of body and soul that followed. Overnight, after an ill-conceived business trip to New York, I became housebound. In the cataclysm of this more serious phase of illness I was finally forced to restructure both my life and identity and to place myself among the CFIDS community, within the continent of the chronically ill.

That hasn't come easily for me. For someone who has had a lifelong antipathy to acknowledging or talking about weakness, "coming out" as a seriously ill person has been a process laden with ambivalence. That I should write about this process seemed, initially, unlikely. In 1997, I had a curious phone conversation with a cousin. Her mother, a beloved aunt, was dying from Parkinson's disease after having suffered for ten years from eosinophilia-myalgia syndrome (EMS), a protracted, painful disease similar to CFIDS caused by a poisoned batch of the sleep aid L-tryptophan. We commiserated and, knowing perhaps of a writer's itch, my cousin asked if I planned to write about what I'd gone through in the last couple of years.

"No way! Let someone else do that." The thought of revisiting those painful days was appalling. I was desperate to return to health, not relive illness.

But that same fall I found myself scribbling notes. An essay took shape, another. Gradually—very gradually—a book cohered. My brain often swam in a fog so thick I could write only a few sentences a day. The combination of fatigue, brain fog, and visual processing problems limited my computer time initially to fifteen or twenty minutes a couple of times a week. By 2004–05, as I finished the book, I was up to an hour or two a day, an absolute bonanza. The biggest challenge was research; I have difficulty holding more than one thought in my head, let alone remembering and organizing a whole body of information. I pasted together ideas one thought, one sentence at a time, putting my finger on the paragraph or quote I wanted to use and integrating it into my text immediately, before the thought evaporated. Many times I felt overwhelmed by the work. Many times I considered abandoning it. But something in me was compelled to turn those months and years into something more than a string of dark days.

I often felt in awe of the biochemical battles and storms, that blustery inner atmosphere of my body, as I lay quiet, at once battleground and observer. For all the exhausted silence of the ill, for all the dismissive silence of the medical community, CFIDS is not a quiet guest. CFIDS has stirred storms among families and patients, government officials, physicians, researchers, insurance companies, media. It has ignited debate and controversy about the very nature of illness, about how illnesses are recognized and defined and who has this power. It has exposed the way medical specialization fragments conversation about the body and revealed the flimsy scaffolding of medical beneficence. CFIDS is a wrench in individual lives, family lives, but also in our culture's concepts of illness and our faith in medical solutions.

"Illness always seems to tell us more about a person or an era than health does, although it is not clear why," writes literary scholar David Morris.[8] This is certainly true of CFIDS, which is not a blip on the medical radar but a sign of flux, in which one story about illness is breaking down and another emerging. Are we witnessing the advent of "postmodern" illness, in which the triumphalism of modern science is brought up short by an upsurge in illnesses that don't readily fit under the rubric of scientific medicine? David Morris and others suggest just that, declaring these enigmatic illnesses to be the "indigestible leftover generated through the binary thinking endemic to western rationalism, a residue in excess of what the biomedical model can accommodate or explain."[9] Postmodern illnesses are messy, complex, multicausal. They won't be conquered in the laboratory alone. They require a holistic approach, taking into account psychosocial and environmental factors. They demand a collaborative effort between patient and doctor, and a keen attention to the patient's subjective experience, not only to test results.

I suspect the tools of bioscience will eventually unravel the enigma of CFIDS—recent microarray technology holds promise of a diagnostic test for CFIDS—but only in part. The mystery of CFIDS and other controversial chronic illnesses cannot be untangled without considering the impact on our immune and nervous systems of an environment flooded with pollutants and chemicals; without examining the way our medical system and public policy support or fail to support the ill; or without listening to the stories of the ill, the discomfiting, day-to-day details that the microscopically focused lens of mainstream medical practice cannot capture and that the healthy in their separate country rarely see.

With this accretion of daily reports of sweat and dizziness and pain, the ill body is brought back from that dark interior landscape George Beard described in the nineteenth century. The growing collection of stories about CFIDS, in all their uncomfortable detail, is what will bring the occulted bodies of those with CFIDS into public view and change the dialogue about illness to include CFIDS in its terms.

In many ways, the CFIDS story is an unsettling roadmap for the illness experience of the future, in which one group of patients is well served by the advances of biomedicine, and another is left behind. In the vacuum created by Western medicine, alternative healers and patient advocacy groups flourish, raising further conflict over medical authority and voice. I wrote this book to illuminate these multilayered struggles and to pull this illness from confusion, obscurity, and distortion, to make it visible.

Encounters
with the Invisible

Listening to Einstein
in the Dark

March 1996

In the evening as we lie in bed, Bill sweeps his palms over the contours of my head and down my spine, along my arms and legs, grazing my skin as if moving over a Ouija board. This has a soothing effect on the muscle pain that clenches my body. He's got the technique down, a touch so light it's like a laying on of hands. Moving *chi*, a friend later tells me. Our improvisation is apparently similar to a technique Chinese healers use to stimulate *chi*, vital energy. *Chi* or not, the radiating warmth of his hands seems to pull some of the pulsing ache from my muscles.

This may seem a tender moment, but it's not. We're sunk in a boggy, tense confusion. I don't know what Bill is thinking. It's dark, and my throat is too sore to talk. His body curved next to mine casts an intimate heat, but I imagine his face has the erased, blank look of someone simply enduring. He strokes my skin because he wants to help, because it's something he can do. Because I've asked him to. He's burdened, exasperated, trying.

It strikes me that our improvised act goes to the heart of this illness, an expressive mime. Trying things in the dark, in silence, without knowing why. Going on instinct because not much else is offered, no remedy or explanation. Borrowing from Eastern techniques because Western medicine has little to say. And discovering that we can, in our own bumbling way, do something that helps, something rooted in the body, of the body, for the body.

Another scene, this one also in bed, since that's where I am now, day and night. I've discovered a technique for "watching" TV with Bill. We switch off the lights, turn the sound as low as possible. Eyes closed, I listen to a documentary or nature show, the ones with the slow, soothing voices that won't overwhelm my addled brain. A few sentences, a pause, a few more sentences in that serene voice meted out in parcels I can manage. MTV in reverse. The aural equivalent of large-print books.

Face pressed into my pillow, soles of my feet clamped against Bill's calf for warmth, I listen one night to a program about Einstein. In the lacunae between sentences I repeat the words in my mind. Without this effort, the words wash over me as unintelligible babble. I strain to make each sentence register, to draw sense out of it, to conjure up its story. I see Einstein in my mind's eye. His wild, white hair, his silent chalked brilliance on the blackboard, his long-suffering wife—why does she put up with him, the fool—stirring his stew in her own silence.

Einstein lives in my brain, chalk dust flying. Only I can't make out his revelations. His equations swim unmoored in a vast, black universe. That's how I imagine them, letters and numbers bloated up large, faded, curved, floating away, uninterpretable and enigmatic. Those essential principles that can explain everything drift away in the dark, disappearing among the gaps and fissures in my head.

An apt image, as it turns out. Many people with CFIDS have what is called focal brain damage, which makes me think of pinholes. MRI (magnetic resonance imaging) brain scans of people with CFIDS often reveal tiny punctate lesions, punctate indicating their pencil-point size, usually in the subcortical white matter. Disconcertingly, these are called UBOs, "unidentified bright objects," since these points appear on the scan as small white spots, casting those of us with CFIDS into a sci-fi dream, which feels fitting.

Like Einstein's, our brains are lit by constellations of brilliant, unfathomable light. Neuroradiologists argue over what these maps of inner light mean. Have the UBOs of inner space always been there, remaining unseen until new technology brought them, literally, to light? Are they found in healthy adults? Or do they mark a pathology that explains to tens of thousands of people with CFIDS why they find themselves disoriented and confused, putting the garbage in the dishwasher or trying to make a phone call with a calculator?

Brain injury. Viral assault to the brain. These terms, frightening though they are, make sense to me. I am injured, impaired. I stand in the shower with no idea how to make the water cooler, which knob to turn which way. I pour milk into the sink instead of my cereal bowl. If I spot my glasses on the bedside table and reach for them, then seeing my water glass, stop to take a drink, I forget all about the glasses. Distracted by one thought, I can't keep another in my head.

When they investigated the Incline Village, Nevada, epidemic that occurred in the mid-1980s, Harvard researcher Dr. Anthony Komaroff and his colleagues found brain lesions in 21 percent of healthy controls, but nearly 80 percent of those who were ill with the mystery disease.[1] These researchers suggested the illness might be a "chronic, immunologically mediated inflammatory process of the central nervous system."[2] Others in the medical community disputed these interpretations.

We're all finding our way in the dark.

1

Encounters with the Invisible

But of all this daily drama of the body there is no record. People write always of the doings of the mind.

—Virginia Woolf, "On Being Ill"

September 1995

If illness begins in a spirit of blindness to what is happening and what is to come, it hurtles forward as a series of forced moments of seeing. Before I knew what lay ahead, the trouble I was getting into, I had two moments of clear, if still partial, vision. The first was on a narrow Berkeley side street of small shingled bungalows as I took my daily walk. It was September 18, a hot late-summer day. Bill matched his stroll to my crawl—I kept tugging his arm to go slower. I had a sharp earache, sore throat. We'd gone three blocks, and I was too weak to go on. I stopped in front of a tiny, haphazard yard sprouting dandelions and leggy yellow tea roses poking over a split-rail fence.

In that way that illness intensifies and distorts experience so that a small detail leaps to attention while worlds of importance are mangled into background static, something about those scraggly roses caught my eye. I don't know what it was, but I was drawn to them with a visceral intensity. I leaned over to take in every detail, each curled and faded petal, the hairy tangle of bristly stamens. They were past bloom, giving off a vinegary tinge behind a high, thin edge of sweetness. Maybe it was their simplicity or ordinariness. Their anchored stillness. Whatever it was, I felt suddenly rooted and washed with sanity. "I don't have to go," I said to Bill. "I don't have to do this. There are other ways to finish the book." I meant the trip to New York I was to take in five days to finish interviews for a book I was under deadline to complete.

A clenching anxiety shot through me when I thought of boarding the plane. I knew I was too ill, the chronic fatigue syndrome I'd had for fifteen years worsening. But I'd already canceled the trip a few months earlier because of my illness. I'd rearranged everything and had an elaborately packed interview schedule, with people coming in from Philadelphia, Boston, upstate New York. I wouldn't be able to line them all up like this a third time. To cancel again would signal some final capitulation, some bodily surrender I couldn't face. We stood for a moment under the white sun, then turned toward home.

I did go. I knew I would. Hope, denial, refusal to give up, recklessness, ignorance, irrationality of the most supreme order—whatever it is that drives us to do the things that pull us to the brink, and over, that force was too strong. Six days later I woke in the Washington Square Hotel in Greenwich Village, in a cramped room with pleated blue curtains unsuccessfully trying to buffer street noise and an air conditioner. Bill—with me for a few days before attending a Latin American Studies conference in Washington, D.C.—had gone for coffee. I crouched on the toilet in the narrow bathroom, queasy, staring at uneven, cracked blue tiles. This was my second moment of lucidity. A terrible feeling swept me, a dread felt as a stomach punch. It was too late. I was very ill and I was in New York, three thousand miles from home, in a strange hotel. The damage was done. With that kind of knowledge that seizes the body, a clutch in the solar plexus, an icy blade of premonition, I knew I was in trouble.

That day and the next two, I forced myself into a cab, swerving through New York traffic to meet each interviewee. Bill came with me, gray fright in his eyes, giving directions, counting the change so I could sink into a closed-eye stupor, oblivious to the rattling New York streets, blaring Broadway marquees. My heaviness worsened, my throat a raw slice, like flesh peeled back. On the third day, with two to go, Bill propped me up in front of the door of an office in an industrial building, then disappeared down the hall to wait. I'd given up on conducting real interviews. I just wanted to meet the people, take a few notes and leave. An hour later I lay down on the flowered bedspread in our hotel room and knew my trip was over. So profound was the weakness that gripped me—it's strange to think of weakness as having force or power, an immobilizing grip, but it does—I could no longer speak.

"Why are you so weak?"

Back in California, I was installed on an exam table in a blind exhaustion, eyes closed to the fluorescent lights above. My body felt pressed against the paper-covered vinyl as if I were on a planet with 2 Gs.

As happens with HMOs, where a different doctor appears in the doorway each time you're there—rather like revolving automatons in one of those old German clocks, I sometimes thought—the doctor who stepped through the door was a woman I'd never seen before. Scrunched into a chair against the wall, Bill had explained in his matter-of-fact lawyerly voice when she came into the room that I had chronic fatigue syndrome and a sinus infection and had just returned Friday from New York quite ill. By Sunday night my sinus infection was so intense I felt poured with concrete, down my face, through my cranium, neck, shoulders, and halfway down my back. I needed more antibiotics—the doctor Bill had rushed me to in New York had given me only a three-day supply.

This was Monday morning. Bill had dropped me at the curb of the medical center, then gone to park. It was only ten yards to the foyer, but each step was increasingly difficult. A syrupy weight ran through my head and limbs, pressing me down, my legs wobbly and rocky, as if I'd just stepped off a boat. The comings and goings of people vibrated around me, distant and confusing. It occurred to me I might not make it to the doctor's office on the third floor. I looked around for a wheelchair and some assistance, but didn't see anything. It seemed easier just to get myself upstairs.

I made it to the elevator, stunned by the growing weakness in my legs, pressure in my chest, as if I had to push against tightly stretched canvas to breathe. On the third floor I sagged. The length of hallway ahead loomed as an impossible distance. I was afraid I might collapse on the floor right there. I thought maybe I should. Bill would find me after parking the car and bring a wheelchair. Dazed, I stumbled woodenly forward. The hallway took on a surreal dimension, elongated and thin. Disorientation narrowed my vision to a downcast blur of my plaid flannel shirt, the blue industrial carpet, each foot stepping in front of the other, as I willed myself in a robotic lurch down that hallway. A woman ahead of me, alarmed, leapt to hold open the heavy glass door. I slid to a chair in the waiting room. When Bill came in he brought me a wheelchair.

The doctor stood on the other side of the exam room, my chart in front of her, and eyed me clinically, clearly suspicious of the wheelchair crowding the small cubicle. She read the notations on my chart. Blood pressure normal. Temperature 99.3. Nothing unusual. Slight sore throat, chest clear. She took my blood pressure again, standing up and lying down. Normal. Took my pulse lying down, then had me stand and laid her fingers on my wrist again. Ah. My pulse raced from the simple exertion of standing.

This gave me a tiny iota of credibility. This was measurable, tangible. But it wasn't enough. Rounding up the usual suspects, she wanted me tested for anemia, thyroid, diabetes. Weakly, I shook my head. I knew all blood tests would come back normal, as they had throughout this illness. I could no more explain to her the last fifteen years of exhaustion, brain fog, chronic sore throat, the catastrophic collapse I had just endured in New York, than I could have given a speech in a lecture hall. I fell back on the crinkly paper of the exam table.

I don't know what this doctor thought about chronic fatigue syndrome. I assume she was simply not knowledgeable, like most doctors at my HMO. I wasn't surprised. I'd long since given up on expecting any physician at my HMO to help me cope with my illness. By 1995 you could find a few physicians who were up-to-date on this illness. Some even advocated for those afflicted with CFS. Increasingly, you could find physicians who were politely tolerant. But there were still plenty of doctors who would peddle backwards on their little wheeled stool and get that tense look on their face when you told them you had CFS: "We know of no organic basis for this illness." Chronic fatigue syndrome was an irritant. It's so blatantly unmedicalized, so subjective, another one of those so-called "functional illnesses," like irritable bowel syndrome, that have always plagued medical practitioners, presenting symptoms with no known cause.

Then there are the psychiatrists, medical historians, journalists, and cultural critics who, throughout the 1980s and '90s, were utterly dismissive of CFIDS. I read their diatribes with an appalled and furious fascination. From the disbelievers there are scathing polemics, a whole literature that dismisses patients as "victims of sensationalist media propaganda and medical charlatanism." There are cries of "vogue diagnosis," "fad." Fact sheets pumped out by advocacy groups documenting biological findings are called "propaganda." The diagnosis of CFS is dismissed as breeding hopelessness. It's impugned as a wastebasket diagnosis, a cover for what is primarily psychological distress.

Skeptical physicians claim we're simply "longing for organicity," as historian Edward Shorter has said, desperate for an organic diagnosis to stave off the stigma of psychological illness (never acknowledging that it's the Descartian mind/body split of a mechanistic Western medicine—if we can't find the problem in your body, it must be in your head—that puts us in this position). In fact, many of these skeptics ask with puzzlement: now that mental illness is understood in organic terms and less stigmatized, why should these people with CFS get so upset about a psychiatric attribution? In 1997, more than a decade after CFS appeared in clusters across the United States, of 147 articles about the illness on Medline, 27 percent ascribed a psychiatric cause.[1] In her 1997 book *Hystories,* feminist theorist Elaine Showalter insisted those with CFS were responding hysterically to media coverage about chronic fatigue syndrome and spurning the treatments they really needed: psychotherapy and antidepressants. Not content with simple aspersions, she lumped us in the same camp as people who claim they've been abducted by aliens, a rather hysterical reaction if ever there was one.[2]

The real travesty of this disregard has only more recently come to light. In the early 1990s the Centers for Disease Control (CDC) estimated the number of people with CFIDS to be between 2 and 10 per 100,000, a figure that immediately came under fire from patient advocacy groups.[3] In part because of their pressure, in 1998 the CDC conducted a prevalence study in Wichita, Kansas, and surrounding Sedgwick County, an area demographically similar to the entire United States. This time, instead of relying on doctors to report the disease (the very doctors who often discounted or failed to recognize this illness), the CDC investigators called 20 percent of the population, asked questions about fatigue, then evaluated in a clinic those who had CFS-like symptoms to determine if they did in fact have CFIDS. When looking at an entire community rather than only those people with access to health care and persistence in obtaining a diagnosis, the researchers concluded that a staggering 183 people per 100,000 have CFIDS, almost twenty times the CDC's highest original estimate.[4]

Psychologist Dr. Leonard Jason of DePaul University and his colleagues had also been suspicious of the early CDC numbers. After conducting a pilot study in 1991, they received funding in 1995 from the National Institute of Allergy and Infectious Diseases (NIAID) to conduct a community-based study in Chicago, Illinois, among an ethnically diverse population.[5] The results of the Chicago study, published in 1999, revealed a prevalence rate of 422 per 100,000, which translates to roughly 800,000 adults in the United States with CFIDS.[6] Even more disturbing, 90 percent of the people in this study who met the established criteria for CFIDS had never been diagnosed. Besides revealing CFIDS as a major public health problem, the Wichita and Chicago studies paint an astounding picture of an invisible community, struggling to maintain lives without the benefit of diagnosis, validation, medical support, or treatment.

I have often wondered how these tens of thousands of people have carried on, wondered how they managed their lives, wondered if their dreams have been filled as mine have with images of dragging the self uphill, hand over hand, the body a dead weight. I imagine they've labored, as I have, to find a language for this illness, words to convey the otherness of their lives. If someone has cancer, we know what that word means: surgery, chemotherapy, radiation, hair loss, weakness, nausea. The name sinks in with sharp, terrifying recognition. If I tell someone I have chronic fatigue syndrome, they're likely to say, "Yeah, I'm tired all the time, too," or "Yeah, my friend had that, but I think she was depressed."

I find myself reaching for analogy: I'm like a car with one piston. My head feels packed with wet sand. Or I make comparisons others can understand. Brain fog is the fatigue you'd feel if you'd been on the computer for twelve-hour workdays two weeks running. My leg muscles ache and pulse, making it hard to go up a flight of stairs, much as yours might if you'd run too far the day before. But these descriptions fall wildly short. It's the fiery amalgam, the painful, incapacitating totality of these individual symptoms with dozens of others, that is CFIDS, something more potent and of another magnitude than the complaints of an essentially healthy person.

I wonder if those thousands of others stumbling through their lives unacknowledged, unseen, have succumbed as I have to the pressure of skepticism and the enticement of normalcy, if they've remained silent in the face of disbelief and ignorance. For all the times I've tried to explain this illness to others, there have been just as many times I felt too tired to make the effort. I often preferred to shoulder the burden of illness in private rather than fight not only illness but the battle for recognition and assistance. It was simpler to go incognito, or to tell people of my illness on a need-to-know basis, than to face the misunderstandings, projections, and well-meaning suggestions of others with little or no knowledge of this illness. When I waded through my day behind a filmy screen of exhaustion, the last thing I wanted was for someone to tell me of the latest cure for fatigue they'd heard of from their neighbor's boyfriend's mother.

Invisibility is luxury as well as burden. As long as I could carry on I could meet the world as teacher, mother, neighbor, not "that person who is ill," the label that can supplant all else. "Passing" as a well person can be an act of self-preservation, allowing dignity, control, and a chance to maintain a pre-illness identity, often vital to one's sense of self. It also increases the invisibility of this illness. And, depending on how ill you are, it can be folly, exacting a cruel price.

A few months before my trip to New York, I slumped into an achy haze as my office door clicked shut behind my departing writing client. There was a brief silence as she descended the carpeted stairs, then the thick slam of the solid street door and the rattling echo of the wooden building. A blue light came through the small northern window of my office. The expanse of white desk—scattered with manila files, ledgers, books studded with Post-its, old invoices, pencils, and paper clips—pulsated with my fatigue. Drained as I was, I'd enjoyed the hour with my client, a bitter and disorganized but hugely talented fiction writer. Colorful scarf thrown over my blouse, dressed for normalcy, I had flung open the office door, pleased to see her. To her grim, "How are you," I had answered firmly, "Fine." I drew on every ounce of energy, as if sucking last drops through a straw, as we parsed her manuscript, phrases about scene construction and authorial voice rolling off my tongue. She never knew I was ill.

Some days I made myself sit in the office for a few minutes so my client wouldn't see me leave right after her, as I made a beeline for home and bed with an ironic speed. That day I hadn't bothered, following her quickly down to the sidewalk, tossing a bright smile her way as she fought with her stacks of papers, huge floppy purse, and the car door, then rounding the corner to my car. I imagined I looked like a busy person off to an appointment or a late lunch before heading back to work. It was too easy to fool people, and too hard. With what desperation I held to the seductive illusion of health, the mask of ordinariness. I was clinging to that old self that was fast floating away, the part of me well enough to get by. I wasn't willing to let that old self go, to say simply, "I'm ill."

As a writer I've always been intrigued with the invisible. Writers are supposed to believe in the ineffable. We struggle to hoist this elusive dimension into view through language, filling pages with worlds never before seen in quite the same way. I didn't yet know I was about to become even more invisible than I'd been, cloistered at home, my public presence gone. Or that in my new invisibility, I would be fully seen as a person with CFIDS.

I went home from the doctor that Monday, October 2, 1995, after the New York debacle, and crawled into bed with the relief of someone back from battle, the imprint of disaster pulsating through my body. All I wanted was pillows and calm. And my antibiotics. My daughter Lisa— living at home after college—placed them in my palm and I gobbled

them down. Then a bowl of vegetable barley soup that she handed me,
her eyes shiny with concern, as I lay curled and disheveled. "I'm messed
up," were my last words before I collapsed into sleep. With a blindness
that staggers me to think of now, I believed that with a couple weeks of
rest, I'd be able to carry on.

2

Seeing

A great deal of the intellectual effort of the last hundred years has been spent visualizing what was once invisible.

—Bettyann Holtzmann Kevles, *Naked to the Bone: Medical Imaging in the Twentieth Century*

October 3, 1995

White walls, skylights, cream-colored Berber carpet. As soon as my eyes open in the morning I'm washed with fresh relief. I have never been so glad to be home, in my own bed, my salmon sheets, beige chenille comforter. This is where I need to be, in a small, familiar space, amid washrags and toast crumbs. "Concentrated is my soul in my molar hole," Freud reportedly said when he had a toothache. He understood the way pain draws in the boundaries of a life.

My body is florid with pain, aches flaming through every muscle. And my head: a flat-iron presses the right side of my face; veins of pressure grip my cranium, as if all the seams of my skull were injected to bursting with some venomous fluid. Thoughts move through resistance, like sound through water. My forehead aches with the effort.

Bill comes into the room, a marooned look on his face. I need to go to the bathroom. I slip my bare legs over the side of the bed, my heart pounding from the exertion, and wait for that elevator feeling to settle, light-headed, dizzy. After a moment I stand, heaviness in my legs, airiness in my head, until my internal atmosphere balances and I can take a few steps. Bill slips his arm around my waist, grasping my elbow. Ow, I cry. The slightest pressure on my skin is painful, as if I've been whacked head to toe with a rubber hose. He lets go his hold, supports me, gingerly, fifteen feet to the toilet, my legs crumpling.

I need enclosure, protection, routine. Mountains of comfort food, steamed potatoes and broiled chicken. Hot compresses that I lay, scalding, across my face. Handfuls of vitamins. I need to be steadied by my accustomed view out the second-story bank of bedroom windows—extravagant Monterey pine, scrims of bamboo, droopy Chinese elm, coppery crown of Japanese maple that thrusts through the deck below, sheds and vines, snatches of gray-shingled roof, a distant tip of fir. The vegetative montage has a reassuring clarity, though looking out the window stings my eyes. I can't tolerate bright light. Ordinary sounds assault my ears. A normal tone of voice is painful. Shh, I beg. Bill's voice hurts, as if I were next to a huge reverberating bell.

He carries upstairs on a bamboo tray a saucepan of steaming water and sets it on a potholder on the white melamine bedside table. We figure out to shove several phone books under the pot so I don't have to bend over as much, my neck and back strung with ropes of pain. I drape a kitchen towel over my head and inhale the thin, curdling steam, trying to loosen the packed mud in my head. This is what my life has come to, I think, small and steamy and shrouded, staring Zen-like into a pot of water. "There was only that pain, only that room," wrote Katherine Anne Porter, ravaged by the flu of 1918.[1]

When, two weeks later, I'm still too weak to navigate my way to the kitchen downstairs, I enlist Lisa to lug the microwave into the bedroom. Bill thinks it'll be a hassle, but she gives me her conspiratorial "don't worry Mom" look and hauls it up. She sets up camp: microwave on the cedar chest under the window, the cooler on a blue towel on the nubby carpet. Each morning she carries in quart-sized plastic yogurt containers of ice before dashing to her job as a waitress, from one wait job to another. Bill stuffs the cooler with soups, chicken, canned peaches. Our

room has become the makeshift encampment of the unsettled, the dis-
placed—littered with brown glass vitamin bottles, saucers of soggy mint
tea bags, green plastic thermos, water mug, tea mug, relaxation tapes,
Sony Walkman, electric heating pad, hot water bottle, Blistex lip balm,
crumb-spattered plates.

I flop in bed in an old green T-shirt torn under one armpit. I pee
into a graying half-gallon plastic container that once held potato salad,
set atop a faded towel at the side of the bed, the prattle of urine jarring
Bill awake at night. We're like refugees huddled in one room, cooking,
eating, sleeping, peeing in the small, disordered space.

Bill lines up doctor appointments, though the thought of going out
is appalling to me, the world a cacophony of noise, commotion, wind. I
put in foam earplugs and cinch a sweatshirt about my head. Bill eyes me
warily as he loads me into the car.

These drives are exhausting. I shut my eyes except for a few fleeting
glimpses. Flashes of gas stations, storefronts, signs, streetlights jog my
brain in a familiar way, but I can barely absorb them. The jostling of the
car rocks me with pain. I can't imagine how people dash about as they
do.

One young physician pats my hand and encourages Bill and me to
go away for a weekend, as if a cool seaside breeze and a couple good
nights of sleep will take care of things. Another suggests I try to get ten
hours of sleep two nights in a row; that always revives him. My own
internist, just back to work after taking a leave for depression, takes in
the wheelchair jammed against a medical supply cabinet, the plugs stuck
in my ears, and affects a magnanimous air. He warms his stethoscope
against his palm and sets it on my chest and back. His voice carries an
encouraging tone. "Why don't you talk to a therapist. It really can help."

"Can you look at my throat?" I croak. It's an inexplicable sore throat,
mild and catastrophic at the same time. A couple of filmy white patches and a swollen purplish vein on my uvula the only evidence. Yet two

words bring a cutting pain, like cracking open a scab, as if I have no mucous membrane, only exposed, raw vocal cords.

He drones on about how much therapy can help, the fact that I can barely whisper an irrelevancy he waves away like smoke. A string of words floats through my head, the words of that woman I used to be, who could explain to him his misunderstanding. But I'm too weak to speak, and the weight of space is a physical pressure on my skin like some etheric mush.

Tori Ellison, an artist who works in mixed media and uses X-ray in her abstract paintings, had a life-imitates-art moment when she learned she had multiple sclerosis. When viewing her own MRIs she said, "I find these records peculiarly fascinating. It is almost as though the X-rays, and other forms of imaging the body, are proof of my own existence, in a way that external images of me and the world are not. Or perhaps they signify a more personal sense of identity, beyond my outward appearance and experience."[2]

Proof of my own existence. These words stop me. Staring at her MRIs, Ellison makes a remarkable leap, elevating technology from something used to diagnose or decipher illness to something with onto- logical powers. One literally comes into being through these visible images of an internal world, as the private and unseen are made public and apparent. Ghostly and partial, these images have the capacity to cre- ate a self, to remold and reshape a vision of who we are.

It may sound like magical thinking to impress medical images with a metaphysical stamp, but Ellison's perceptions ring with a peculiar truth. As a person with CFIDS, I know the power of technology to bring a person into existence—or not. It is precisely the power of these lumi- nous scientific images to offer "proof of existence" that creates for peo- ple like me such problems. Without some medically accepted, visible pathology, we remain in that gray area of medical doubt and suspicion.

As one CFIDS patient put it, "The difference between a crazed neurotic and a seriously ill person is simply a test."[3] Ellison's fascination with these powerful images is tempered for me by thoughts of their arrogant use, as science raises to an almost mystical reverence the tangible, physical, seeable.

Technological medicine, it seems, is all about seeing. Not just ordinary seeing, but the audacity and power, even thrill, of seeing into hidden vistas. For all their technical aridity, high-tech machines are instruments of the senses, whose visual reach has rendered the human body more probed and peered into than at any time in history. It's easy to forget how resistant the body has been throughout history to visual penetration. In the late 1800s many physicians were beginning to send specimens of urine, blood, feces, or sputum to the lab as an inroad to the body, but the view of those internal regions—glossy liver, slippery coils of intestine, ducts and vessels—remained a death view, exercised on a cadaver.

Then in 1885 German physicist Wilhelm Roentgen stunned the world with his accidental discovery that cathode rays could penetrate skin to make visible the bones within. Those first ghostly outlines of the skeletal bones of Frau Roentgen's hand—her wedding ring a dark orb floating on a stick of white—became an overnight sensation from Europe to America. Roentgen's discovery of what he called "a new kind of light" opened an unprecedented, previously unthinkable view into the human body.[4] Ever since, increment by increment—with CT scans, MRI, ultrasound, electron microscopy, functional MRI, PET scans—the body has surrendered its mysterious opacity.

This ability to defy the opaque body has had a profound impact on how we think about illness. Enamored of our power to scrutinize and define disease at the anatomic or physiologic level, we increasingly legitimize disease by its physiological evidence. Many diseases, such as hypercholesterol or hypertension, are now defined solely on the basis of a measurable physiologic abnormality, whether or not a person has symptoms. And diseases that used to be diagnosed by a patient's report of symptoms are now defined by test results, such as a white blood count or electrocardiogram.

Internist Robert Aronowitz gives the example of a patient with chest pain who was told he did not have angina pectoris because tests ruled out myocardial infarction and clogged arteries. Before these diagnostic tests became available, the patient would have been diagnosed as having angina pectoris simply on the basis of his symptoms. "Changing disease definitions," writes Dr. Aronowitz, "often reflect compelling beliefs in transition and/or conflict. In this case, a priority given to the way a disease is experienced by a patient is in conflict with the belief that a specific, measurable, and visible abnormality is the best way to define disease."[5]

High-tech instruments do more than give us an inside view; they change our basic concept of disease. Definitions of disease have always involved a complex interplay among patients, physicians, prevailing social and medical beliefs, even legal and governmental interests. Medical instruments are one more player, and an increasingly powerful one. The marvelous ability to watch a T-cell attack a tumor cell or to track the blood flow in a particular region of the brain shapes medical thinking and has an unexpected, often unrecognized side effect. These technologies create a hierarchy of patients, with those at the top, who can brandish clear evidence of disease, graced by medical acceptance, and those at the bottom who can't, tainted by medical distrust. For the patient, our technological abilities to illuminate interior space can be a saving grace (when we detect a cancer early, chances of cure often improve) or an excuse for disregard and dismissal. These instruments can provide "proof of existence" or erase us from view.

This is where things get tricky. In matters medical, as in other matters, seeing isn't a clear-cut enterprise. Identifying a physical abnormality is much more fraught and tenuous than those imposing, high-tech machines suggest. To begin with, even those revealing radiologic images or laboratory tests are subject to error, interpretation, and misreading. No one has successfully stripped the lab of its human element. But beyond that, what you see depends on what you look for, and what your instruments readily reveal. And if you're studying a disease you think important—cancer, Alzheimer's—you're going to look a lot harder for those abnormalities and demand more money for research than you will in the case of a disease entity you question.

Consider this: a remarkable 1994 study by Dr. Anthony Komaroff of Harvard Medical School and his colleagues compared SPECT scans of depressed people, people with AIDS dementia, CFIDS patients, and controls.[6] The findings? The brains of those with CFIDS look remarkably similar to those with AIDS dementia and quite different from those of depressed patients or controls. Years later, when I examine the published article, I'm caught between a gasp of alarm and an exhalation, a letting out of breath that comes with each hint of comprehension.

The brain scans of a control subject show a walnut-shaped cross-section in a psychedelic, computer-enhanced rainbow of color. A thin cordon of wavy purple runs around the rim. Nested inside are undulating thicknesses of magenta and orange with embedded pockets of bright yellow and white, indicating the highest level of brain activity. In the interior cavities, like the meat in a walnut, is more wavy purple spotted with small islands of black. The meat part of the walnut is small; the bright, colorful areas are thick and substantial. The whole is vivid, sturdy, showing no abnormalities.

By contrast, the SPECT scans of those with AIDS dementia and CFIDS are like a city whose lights have been dimmed. The outline of purple has thickened; the areas of magenta and orange have become islands, reduced, thinned-out, or missing altogether. There are only a few small spots of yellow or white. Large globular islands of black fill the interior space. Called "multiple perfusion defects," these are places where blood flow is low and the brain isn't getting the energy it needs to function.

There's a frightening, almost ghoulish vacancy to these images, with their empty pools of black and sketchy, reduced areas of activity. How can these people function? Is this why I can't do two things at once, why I'm overwhelmed by noise and activity, why I can't remember the word for oatmeal? Are these the biological tracings of my confusion, some inner blankness shutting down that old, vital self?

Part of me resists the thought of being set alongside those with AIDS dementia, when, in the final stages of the disease, the AIDS virus in the brain begins to stamp out language, memory, mental clarity. "Wally begins to have trouble finding the words he wants," remembers poet Mark Doty in his searing memoir of his lover's death from AIDS. "We're lying in bed talking about something and he says, 'Oh, I'm going to mush my mouse.' Then he looks puzzled. 'Mush my mouse? Oh, what's happening to me!'"[7]

Then I think of how many times I've had moments like that—saying, "I'm out of eager" when I mean "energy," or "Could you hand me the restaurant?" when I mean "washcloth"—and those scans make a scary kind of sense. The scans of the depressed patient in the study, ironically, are much brighter and closer in appearance to those of the control, with far more thick bands of color, much smaller islands of black. Except for a small blank spot, shown as a dark indentation in the left lateral frontal and temporal lobes, the brain of the depressed patient appears normal.

The authors note that the findings on SPECT, those black absences, aren't specific to CFS, appearing in patients with systemic lupus erythematosus, cocaine abuse, and multiinfarct dementia. So these findings aren't useful for diagnosis, but may provide insight into the various underlying disease processes. "The findings in CFS are consistent with the hypothesis that CFS also [like AIDS dementia complex] results from viral infection of neurons, glia, or vasculature."[8]

This study is only one of hundreds of neuroimaging and neuroendocrine studies of CFS patients that now exist, the great majority of which show more abnormalities of the central nervous system in CFIDS patients than in healthy controls. That these abnormalities could result in the symptoms patients experience, says Dr. Anthony Komaroff, "seems to me as indisputable."[9] Why do these studies continue to be ignored, dismissed, or challenged? (One physician I saw in 1996 snorted and called the science on CFS "pitiful.")

The answer lies in the pervasive attitude that CFIDS is primarily psychological in origin, which has plagued this illness from its inception, and the resulting bureaucratic disregard and lack of funding. Hillary Johnson's revealing book, *Osler's Web: Inside the Labyrinth of the Chronic Fatigue Syndrome Epidemic,* chronicles how the Centers for Disease Control and Prevention (CDC) and the National Institutes of Health (NIH) resisted legitimizing this illness, how the politics of research funding prevented investigation, and how the physicians who did take CFIDS seriously were ridiculed and ostracized. She paints a dramatic picture of the way "the bias of federal scientists and their bureaucratic machinations compounded to erase the epidemic from public view."[10]

Adding to an already tawdry story, in the 1990s, patient advocacy efforts exposed an outrageous funding scandal that makes the grand undertakings of the CDC appear less than beneficent. Beginning in the late '80s, Hillary Johnson and others inside and outside the CDC became suspicious that funds appropriated by Congress for CFS research were being used for other purposes.[11] Ms. Johnson undertook a vigorous investigative effort to uncover this misconduct, issuing

Freedom of Information Act requests and talking with people at the CDC and in Congress. By the early '90s the CFIDS Association of America, the largest patient advocacy group for CFS, was also raising questions about how federal CFS monies were being spent. They, too, issued FOIA requests and began pressuring the CDC to detail its spending. Finally, in the summer of 1998, even Dr. William Reeves, the CDC's program director for CFS, could see that money allocated for CFS was being misspent. He blew the whistle on his own agency, and in response, the Inspector General of the Department of Health and Human Services conducted an official audit.

The Inspector General's report, released on May 12, 1999, revealed that between 1995 and 1998 the CDC spent $12.9 million that had been earmarked for CFIDS on other projects, and misled Congress about these funds.[12] According to the report, the CDC had inflated its figures of CFS spending in testimony to Congress by as much as 48 to 72 percent each year. Many patient advocates felt these were conservative figures. Hillary Johnson knew from her investigative work that the problem had begun far earlier, and the CFIDS Association claimed that the "CDC has consistently and intentionally misrepresented its CFS research spending since at least 1991."[13]

The misused funds from 1995–98 have now been restored, mostly in fiscal years 2002 and 2003, but the CFS funding siphoned away for other CDC programs before 1995 will never be replaced, and the many years of unfunded research have seriously compromised the scientific effort to understand CFS. Even with the restored money, federal funding remains appallingly inadequate. In 2003, more than twenty years after the first CFIDS patients, myself included, began straggling into medical offices, the total federal expenditure for CFS research—from both the NIH and CDC—was still a paltry $16 million.[14] By contrast, according to its own documents, the NIH alone spent $99 million on multiple sclerosis in 2003, an illness affecting half as many people.[15] The research conducted in the first fifteen years of the CFIDS epidemic relied primarily on small grants, often funded by patient advocacy organizations or individuals, and necessarily involved small numbers of subjects. To dismiss CFS research as "pitiful" obscures the CDC's malfeasance, betrayal of trust, and glaring absence of attention to a widespread and serious illness.

Since most CFIDS patients show normal results on standard blood tests, medical visibility also depends on physicians knowing about and ordering the less commonly used blood tests that would reveal abnormalities. Over the years, in a pointless ritual, I've periodically rolled up my sleeve and proffered my blood to obliging technicians. The lab results are as predictable as the seasons. Everything normal.

Or is it? Dr. David Bell, a clinician and researcher specializing in pediatric CFIDS, has studied orthostatic intolerance and blood volume in persons with CFIDS (PWCs), and believes that a reduction of blood flow to the brain is a key element of this illness. In 1995, he and the late David Streeten, then a professor of medicine at the State University of New York Health Science Center, Syracuse, used a test not included in standard blood work to reveal low plasma volume (the fluid in blood) and low red blood cell mass. "It's very unusual to do the red blood cell mass test," says Dr. Bell, describing the chromium 51 technique performed in the nuclear medicine department.[16] With standard blood work, low blood volume will not be apparent. "It's impossible to see," he explains. "You can't measure that on a simple blood test from the arm, because the blood, when you take it out in a tube, is perfectly normal blood. It's just that the whole body doesn't have enough of it.

"We don't know why this occurs," he goes on to say. "But when you have a low blood volume to start with, when you stand up, a quart of blood goes down into your legs and you have even less blood going up into your brain."[17] The result? Your brain doesn't get enough oxygen and you're wiped out if you try to engage in normal physical and mental activity.[18]

Barry Hurwitz, Ph.D., professor at the Behavioral Medicine Research Center/VA Medical Center in Miami, is the principal investigator, with immunologist Nancy Klimas, for a study at the University of Miami to see if Procrit can help CFIDS patients. The medication, often used for patients undergoing chemotherapy, works to increase the production of oxygen-carrying red blood cells. Like Drs. Bell and Streeten, Dr. Hurwitz believes low blood volume may help explain the abnormal fatigue CFIDS patients experience. "If you have diminished red blood cell volume, then you have less capability to deliver oxygen to the cells. There's a high probability that if we're able to increase red blood cell volume it will diminish fatigue."[19] He and his colleagues have found that 60 percent of females and 15 percent of males with CFS have low-normal or below-normal red blood cell volume, a finding "usually missed by standard blood tests."[20]

Another example: Many people with CFIDS have an abnormal form of RNase-L, an enzyme that is part of the body's antiviral defense system, raising the possibility of a biomarker for a subset of people with CFIDS. This abnormal RNase-L indicates immune system dysregulation, and a number of studies have correlated it with increased fatigue, lower aerobic function, muscle aches, and cognitive difficulties.[21] But most U.S. physicians don't know about and don't order the blood test, developed in Belgium, that reveals RNase-L abnormalities, and most local labs would be confused by the strange pelletization of blood samples that is required.

Even if doctors knew to order these tests, in this age of managed care, most insurance companies wouldn't cover them. Physician ignorance, lack of funding, lack of insurance coverage—all create a false invisibility. Says patient activist Peggy Munson, "I think the situation of

CFIDS patients is akin to that of death row inmates who are suddenly pardoned due to DNA technology. What is 'seen' in biomedicine changes all the time, and guilt or innocence can hinge on the limits of technology, or the hubris about technology."[22]

I'd go further: overreliance on lab tests and visible pathology is itself the problem. When did we so subdue the ambiguity and complexity of biology as to be able to determine disease legitimacy by tests and scans alone? What happened to the kind of seeing that goes on when the doctor looks at the patient, not only the MRI? What happened to clinical knowledge and intuition, and attention to individual suffering, the great hallmarks of pretechnological medicine?

The fear first expressed in the late nineteenth century, as laboratory science began its ascendancy ("laboratory training *unfits* a man for his work as a physician," wrote Sir James Mackenzie in 1918, bemoaning the loss of focus on the patient), finds new fodder in our molecular, high-tech age.[23] In the name of seeing more, do we see less? Seeing the body piecemeal in the lab—an enzyme, a right temporal lobe—we eclipse the patient, that complex person perched on the exam table.

I hold no romantic view of prescientific medicine. Who would want to return to the days when a catastrophic 29 percent of women giving birth in a hospital might die of puerperal fever—as was the case at Vienna General Hospital in the 1840s—or when antibiotics were an unimaginable dream? But at least back then, when a physician percussed the chest of a patient—most often in that person's home—he regarded the patient's report of chest pain and dizziness as central to his diagnosis.[24] His eye was on the person, not a computer screen. Diagnosis was much more a negotiation between patient and physician. In those prescientific days, before the medical gaze narrowed to the microscopic,[25] the medical humanist Sir William Osler (1849–1919) aptly noted, "The good physician treats the disease but the great physician treats the patient."[26]

Patients are not the only ones dismayed by a "body-snatching" technological medicine. Many physicians grumble about sacrificing the art and intuition of clinical medicine to the strictures of managed care and the laboratory "truths" of biomedicine. Individual doctors and researchers often hold finely nuanced views of disease and compassionate, open-minded readings of a patient's distress. Yet for all but the most renegade of doctors, clinical observation remains hinged to a standard medical practice informed by the revelations of the lab, not the anomalous voice of the body. Diagnosis based on observation and deduction but not backed by organic findings remains controversial, considered unscientific and unsubstantiated.

CFIDS patients have a curious, ambivalent relationship with technology—applauding its successes, believing in its power, demanding its resources, and wary of its limits. On the one hand, as disenfranchised patients, we want access to the realm of scientific cures. We believe that with enough focus and resources the biological mechanism behind CFIDS will be duly revealed and all of us who have suffered the ignominy of disbelief will be granted legitimate standing in the halls of medicine. On the other hand, we have an uneasy feeling—whether under the aegis of a mystic antimaterialism, a fear of medical dominance, or a postmodern indeterminacy—that scientific medicine has narrow tools and narrow minds and can never reduce the complexity of biology to the controlled, so-called "objective" findings of the lab. We're in the confusing position of struggling to be received into technology's graces, while recognizing that the shrine of technology is a complicated altar.

Artist Tori Ellison, observing her ghostly MRIs, was right to intuit their ontological power to call an ill person into being—a power that both aggrandizes scientific medicine and, in the case of someone like myself, betrays its limits. I find myself looking over her shoulder at those eloquent images of the body's mysterious workings, its failures and glitches. How haunting they are, those films of the brain's disarray, dense with significance. What Ellison probably saw in her films were the plaques or lesions in the brain that characterize multiple sclerosis (MS). They appear as bright spots on an MRI, and people with CFIDS have them too—remember those UBOs?—though the lesions of people with MS tend to be ovoid rather than punctate and are more frequently seen in the periventricular regions rather than the subcortical white matter, as is the case for CFIDS.[27]

Do I have those punctate lesions in my brain? I don't know. But I know what I feel, and I know that what I feel should matter as much as technical data. I know that biomedicine needs to accommodate suffering that doctors can't explain or that isn't instantly linked to organic abnormalities. It needs to recognize its limits, its uncertainties, its fallibility. It needs to acknowledge the cultural and technological factors that influence the way we think about and classify disease. It needs to affirm that the observations of the clinic, not just the investigations of the lab, can lead to new knowledge. And it needs to expand medical training to retain the best of nineteenth-century medicine, its strong clinical focus. Dr. David Bell, who treated a cluster of patients with CFIDS in Lyndonville, New York, in the 1980s, says with a hint of wistfulness, "If I were to make any suggestions for changes in American medical schools, it would be that they train doctors to be more like doctors in the nineteenth century. They were great clinicians, and I think they would have handled chronic fatigue syndrome quite nicely."[28]

If the instruments we've developed were as omnipotent as their transcendent gaze suggests—rendering the opaque body obsolete, conferring an authority previously accorded alchemists, shamans, or gods—we'd be in fine shape. Of course they're not. Perhaps we simply expect too much. Sometimes I think of scientific advance as a bravura performance that goes on in one brilliantly lit theater while all the other theaters in town are dark.

3

Silence

I sometimes think that silence can kill you. . . . I think that language, speech, stories, or narratives are the most effective ways to keep our humanity alive. To remain silent is literally to close down the shop of one's humanity.

—Anatole Broyard, *Intoxicated by My Illness:*
And Other Writings on Life and Death

November 1995

After four weeks in bed I slip into silence. The smudge-pot in my throat with its peculiar blend of smoky abrasion, heat, and razor-nicks of pain hasn't eased. I can whisper a few sentences, but more than that makes my throat worse. And the effort of talking is exhausting, crimping my chest and drawing on a strength I no longer have. When Bill ferries in my oatmeal, I mime that I need paper and pen. He stands before me, scratch paper held out with distrust, as if he were colluding in my derangement. I start writing notes, short cryptic phrases, the surface of illness. "I want more of that soup with noodles and chicken. None? Some broth. What else is there? I'm hungry." (I'll amass five hundred pages in the next year before my voice returns, testimony to the clamor of silence.)

There's a lot of bedside sitting and concerned-face making. A friend plants herself on my lumpy quilt and encourages me to talk about what I'm feeling, as if to guide me through the snarled thicket of my fears, as if I just need to work them through. "Can you describe it?"

I blanch, scratch a terse note and shove it at her. "I can't talk! It hurts."

Bill's and Lisa's faces orbit around me, blank and fearful. My silence seems to silence them, in that odd way that the weak and vulnerable exert unspoken leverage over the strong. They don't know what to do, how to help. When I scribble, "I'll do steam. Can you get more vitamins?", they leap into action, relieved to have a task.

"Silence is the greatest cry," says a character in the Holocaust film *Life Is Beautiful*. And indeed, my silence seems to be a siren call that everyone is bent on investing with all sorts of meaning, mostly grave. What a powerhouse of primal emotion silence is. I remember poet Maya Angelou's story of going mute after she was raped at age eight. In the face of her wounding, words had become flimsy, insubstantial, unable to contain or convey what had happened. This kind of silence is its own language, both erasing and insisting on what is too painful to speak. It appears as a defection from the world, an abnegation, withdrawal, but often sustains a fiercely protected life.

Then there's the silence that initiates rest, renewal, restoration. The silence of rejuvenating retreat. The silence that is nourishing, that builds strength and prepares the self for reemergence. "A pregnant pause," "a loaded silence"—these phrases capture the potentiality in silence, its transformative possibilities.

I can say this about silence. It matters. It's never undertaken lightly. It may seem dramatic, but for me it is simply practical. It hurts to talk. I need to shut down, to let my throat heal. Silence is a measure of extremity, of how far removed I am from normal, daily life, from the ease and spontaneity of ordinary exchanges. Removed from a physical place in the world. Removed from language. Shrunk to a small lump in the bed. I seem to have devolved to an elemental state of mottled, primitive expression. Silence. Pain. Hunger.

My new silence doesn't frighten or startle me. I know I can get through this. I'm used to silence, used to my throat giving out for days, even weeks, at a time. Used to the stubborn public silence around this illness, used to my own chosen silence in the face of daily aches, brain fog, and sore throats. This illness itself exists as a silence, a gap in the medical conversation. But I'm unprepared for the new magnitude of this silence I'm entering. I'm unprepared for the way these past years of silence—mine, the medical profession's—and their cargo of misconceptions will come to haunt me when I most need understanding and support. I'm not yet aware of the far reaches this silence will tow me to, an isolated place more distant than the one I already know.

I keep on my bedside table a photo of me, Bill, and Lisa taken at a friend's wedding in June of 1995, just months before my ill-fated trip to New York. We look happy, our faces turned to the camera with broad, relaxed smiles, radiating pleasure. Bill hoists a wine glass, as if life were full and good. We clasp each other around the waist and shoulders.

There's no doubt in that photo, no disarray. The joyful moment is arrested, uncontaminated by the tatters of daily life, the surface wiped clean. I stare at it every day, feeling a rather desperate attachment. I need to believe that is who we are, the three of us, that joined, glowing triptych. That woman in her shimmering green blouse and sparkly necklace—even her eyes sparkle, such amazing aliveness. That is who I am, I tell myself, who I will be again, the person I'm returning to as I heal.

It's fitting that what orients and reassures me is a picture. A static moment, cleansed of context. A wordless moment, an instant preserved in silence behind glass. Much as I long for words, for the connection they bring, there is something about this illness—about any severe illness or misery—that is beyond words. Even if I could speak, what would I say? What words could bring the affinity that arises from shared experience? William Styron, maestro of language, presents a searing account of his near-suicidal descent into depression in *Darkness Visible*, yet declares his words an inadequate shadow of something "indescribable." Ultimately, pain is deeply private. At the moment we most need connection, we are most enclosed in a personal world, scribbling out our fragmented notes like reports from someplace faraway.

"Terrible it is, beyond words' reach," cries Philoctetes, Sophocles' character who has an excruciating wound that will not heal. "Resistance to language," writes professor of English Elaine Scarry in her classic work *The Body in Pain*, is at the very essence of pain, "essential to what it is."[1] Its unsharability, its insular nature, is at its core. Pain inherently carries "this absolute split between one's sense of one's own reality and the reality of other persons."[2] There it is again, that idea of remove, of being split off from others and deposed to a realm of one's own. The breach of language created by pain broadcasts a breach of experience that is a stinging marker of illness, another source of distress.

From my second-story bedroom window I look down on our bamboo-enclosed backyard garden and rectangular studio, a converted garage Lisa has made into her "pad," where she's half at home, half in her own place. Lights blare through the slatted blinds and a bank of clerestory windows along the garden-facing side. Through them I glimpse a triangular slash of the far corner of her room scattered with papers, laundry, fuzzy slippers, a black leather backpack. Afternoons and evenings, she lugs around huge trays of beer mugs and sandwiches at Raleigh's, a student pub on Telegraph Avenue, then hangs out with friends, traveling the city to parties and late-night bar-hopping. For all her devotion to me, she's tethered only lightly to our home.

This evening she's impatient. She's forgotten she promised to stay with me while Bill goes to his Spanish class. I need her presence to combat the frightening feelings of vulnerability that well up when I'm alone.

"Mo-om," she flicks her long hair over her shoulder. An impatient energy ripples beneath her skin. A dancer in college, she's thin and muscled under her baggy U.C. Santa Barbara sweatshirt, lithe and elastic in her movements.

I scribble a note in a shaky hand, the words snaking around the edge of the page filled with other loopy scratchings. "I'm so weak I can barely walk or talk. My chest hurts. I just need you to stay with me in case I need anything. Thanks, sweetie. I love you."

She agrees to one hour of TV, a compromise, and plunks herself, restless, into the curved-beechwood lounge chair next to my bed, shoulders tugged in.

My illness, to her, is a rope to a home she chafes to leave. Or more precisely, to a mother who appears just a bit too redolent of everything she's trying to shake loose from: constriction, confusion, a jarring vulnerability. She's been trying to decide whether to go to graduate school in social work and was unspooling her thoughts to me last week when her eyes suddenly sharpened and I could see her appraising me as if an electric arc had just fired between this image of mother before her and the appalling idea that social work could mean, well, more of the same, as if I were an inopportune avatar of what could lie ahead.

Like everyone, she doesn't understand why I'm so sick, why there isn't something I can do to get better, how much longer this is going to go on, what it will do to her life. She's worried, frustrated, torn. And we can't talk, as we always have, this daughter of mine whose Saturday morning habit for years has been to wander into my room in her pajamas for her partying recap: where she went the night before, with whom, what so-and-so said, what she thought about what so-and-so said, what she said, why they went to this party, not that, why the party was bunk, and on and on until I gently suggest I have some work to get done.

Yesterday she'd wanted to tell me about her new boyfriend, a pink and blond Catholic boy from U.C.S.B. who seems sweet on her—he'd driven up from Santa Barbara to see her last weekend. I'd listened as much as I could. But after a while that sinking fatigue took me, and I couldn't keep my eyes open or my head nodding in response. She'd stalked off.

"All cures are partly 'talking cures,' to use Freud's phrase," said writer Anatole Broyard, dying of cancer.[3] So much for us. My notes to her are repetitive messages for more tea, or ice for the cooler, or an errand I need her to run, or laundry I need retrieved from the rack downstairs. I'm too weak, in too much pain to deal with her confusion. At least she's twenty-three, not sixteen, not twelve. For that, I'm grateful. As soon as the TV program is over, she's off to her rendezvous, her friends.

The next night Lisa comes in before work, trailing the flowery scent of *Anais anais.* She takes up that ubiquitous bedside stance, legs crossed, handing me her own note—funny how my silence snuffs out everyone's voice like a candle cup.

"To be this seriously sick (bed-ridden) for this long—you should see a specialist. I feel selfish when I get pissed off because this is infringing on my life, but I didn't mind doing this for the last month—I wanted to help you—but now a month later to be with the same symptoms you were a month ago, not wanting to be alone—it frustrates me because this has gone on too long. I'm really busy right now, and am trying to live my life—and I can't seem to move forward because I don't have the time and I have to keep putting things off. I'm just frustrated because I feel like at this point we should have moved farther (health-wise)/ you should be able to walk downstairs without feeling so weak. That's why I really think it's unavoidable for you to see a doctor. Trust me. It will be helpful. I love you, too."

We all seem to be exploding with unspoken words. How urgently everyone wants me to revive. One of my sisters has suggested to Lisa that I go to a support group (!). Another sister—I have four—writes a note urging me to try Ayurvedic medicine, and to think about Bill and Lisa, how long can I expect them to take care of me like this? No one can fathom a flulike illness that doesn't resolve in a matter of weeks, that goes on and on and has no cure. My scrawled responses are weak, ineffectual, telegraphed.

At this moment I need words intensely. I know running to doctors is futile, and too much for me. I know I have to listen to my body and stay quiet. I know all the years of illness have dragged my body to a level of debilitation no one comprehends. It's as if I had been five feet down a deep hole to begin with, and now I've fallen to ten feet below ground. No one knew how far down I was, and now they can't see how long it will take to dig myself out. (Nor can I; I still think it will be a matter of months.)

The words that could explain run through my head in muffled chords. That even my daughter doesn't understand fills me with frustration and pain, a sense that I've been lost to the eyes of others.

There's a lethal side to silence. When language is inadequate or unavailable, experience disappears, becomes unseen and unacknowledged. Silence = Death, AIDS activists say, equating silence with annihilation. If those with AIDS don't speak up, don't demand public recognition and the resources to fight their illness, they will literally die. For me the fear is not death but a more subtle annihilation, the slow fade into anonymity. To have to leave the intricacies of this disabling illness unarticulated, unexplained, is to become once again invisible. It is to once again shove the knowledge of my body's disarray underground. It is to have to retreat into monkish quiet when angered by misconceptions. To have to close the door, for now anyway, on all the rages and turbulence this illness creates because I haven't the strength to do otherwise. Without expression and the understanding and alliance it brings, I'm forced into a submitting/defying silence and consigned to a small, insular world.

So to be stripped of voice is a wound in itself. It's interesting that physical pain in literature, when it is presented at all, is often conveyed as a scream. Think of the three-day-long, despairing death wail of Ivan Ilych in Tolstoy's "The Death of Ivan Ilych," or the agonized screams of Sophocles' wounded warrior Philoctetes, one of literature's great vocalists of physical pain. I think, actually, that silence is close kin to those shrieks of pain, speaking of experience at the edge. Silence, too, is a blank, unnuanced caterwaul of the body.

I read Sophocles' play *Philoctetes* with a fascination born of empathy and repulsion: Philoctetes is an awfully self-pitying fellow, ravaged by suffering, swinging wildly between anguish and lust for revenge. His story is fired with bitterness and vengeance. Sailing with the Greek army to Troy to avenge the kidnapping of Menelaus's wife Helen by the Trojan Paris, Philoctetes is felled, bitten by a snake on the island of Chryse. He's left with a vile, hideous wound that, inexplicably, will not heal.

The Greeks abandon Philoctetes on the island of Lemnos because "He kept filling the whole camp with his wild shouts and screams, offending the gods."[4] (Ah, the ease of displacement, blaming the gods.) Unable to bear the sounds of his suffering, the Greeks leave him to survive on his own. This is another truth about pain, the difficulty we, as listeners, have in hearing it. There's such resistance to the tragic moment, such a need to erase or overcome it, to wipe it from view— especially pain that doesn't end, a wound that doesn't heal.

Left to his island with his hideous wound, Philoctetes can only cry in torment: "A, a, a, a!"[5] At the moment the expression of pain is most pure and undeniable, it is the most monotone and emptied of individuality. No longer the expression of an individual but a condition, pain's personal signature becomes undecipherable, clotted into a generic note of anguish. Philoctetes' wild screams are a foreign language, with a meaning at once indisputable and incomprehensible, much like silence.

I remember being struck, when reading a biography of the English poet Christina Rossetti in graduate school, by the noise of her poems—

they clang with tumultuous energy—and the noise of her final painful days. In the evenings, in the weeks and months before she died of cancer in 1894, alone in her London home, she was heard screaming in agony. The language of pain may be preverbal, but it is volcanic. Distressed by her cries, a young neighbor with children wrote Rossetti's brother, pleading with him to do something to erase the sounds of pain, so she and her family wouldn't have to listen to this terrible noise, especially the children. (It's either the gods or the children.) She wanted the sounds of physical pain muted, silenced. She couldn't bear to hear them.

More than a century later and a continent away, I'm disturbed by the thought of those cries. That they were released only when Rossetti was alone, that she kept this most primal expression to herself, or tried. That others didn't want to hear her. That she no longer had the strength to funnel her personal pain into literature. In the throes of her suffering, Rossetti had already fallen beyond the realm where language mattered. She had already reached that absolute habitation of body in which the common tools of speech are rendered useless. This seems the saddest to me: that for a poet so devoted to language, in the end her pain should have overwhelmed her words (the escape into literature is the dodge *into* language, away from those primitive cries), that she had come to a place where language stopped.

I don't like to think this about language, that it can fail me, fail us. Maybe it's not so much that there is no language, as that access to language is closed down. The storms of the body blank out language. The vocabulary of pain is preverbal, full of shrieks and squawks and roars and silences. In pain, we slide away from language, and to reclaim our self is to move back to that place where we can speak.

"This is what it must be like to be dying," I say to Bill one afternoon. He's cradling my forearms, one arm supporting my back as he helps me to the bathroom. Through the bedroom window, leafy greens—

emerald, lime, olive, silvery—glimmer in the sun. They seem remote and apart, their luster and warmth a world I once knew but can no longer reach.

I know I'm not going to die. But I'm visiting that bleak, consuming place where illness skitters frighteningly close to the rituals of impending death. Life as I have known it is gone. All the motions that absorb my day—calls to the doctor, herbs, medications, hot compresses, steam, meditation tapes, soups—are from the world of the ill. Every moment is focused on finding some small relief from pain, a more comfortable position, steam, another teaspoon of viscous decongestant. And every moment is suffused with that torpor and loss of function that have plucked me unequivocally out of the life I had.

This weakness that renders me helpless and dependent is what, more than anything, fills me with fear. I stand briefly in the doorway to Bill's office, two steps from the bathroom. On the far side of his room a casement window overlooks the street. I would love to see the view up our block, the placid bungalows of our neighborhood and their flowering yards. But I can't cross a room without that swooning feeling, my knees going to jelly under me. If only I could do that, I think. Just that— walk across a room and feel ordinary.

There are more indignities: sores on my tongue, gums, and the roof of my mouth that make it difficult to eat. Some strange arrhythmia in my brain that jerks me awake at all hours of the night. I toss down glasses of brown powdered herbs in warm water that lull me into a sedated drift, but through long hours of darkness, unable to sleep, I listen to the distant whir of traffic on Highway 24, the sound of nostalgia and loneliness. And I have increasing weakness in my arms. Sipping soup in bed one morning I realize I'm having trouble holding the glass bowl, cupped in a frayed yellow potholder. My left bicep cramps with thin darts of pain and weakness. Both my arms are weakened, but I'm losing the use of my left arm in particular. A few days later, I can't hold even a piece of paper without feeling a needled, contractive pain in my bicep, as if I've lifted weights way beyond my capacity, the muscle exhausted. Finally I can't use my left arm at all, it hangs slack by my side. These new symptoms in my arms wax and wane, some days worse, some days better.

As the weeks tick off, I'm astounded that I'm unable to get back to work. Last spring I'd come home quite ill after a trip to Costa Rica—travel, obviously, not what I should be doing. It took me five months to recover from the flare-up, but I was back in my office and going out with friends after just a week. Now I can barely manage a shower every other day. One morning, I set a task for myself to file my nails. I have the strength to finish one hand. That's it for the day.

Bill's low voice comes through from his office, adjacent to our bedroom, talking to my friend Sherrie on the phone. He gives a nervous laugh, trying for levity. "I don't know. We're trying not to think about that." I know Sherrie has voiced that unspoken anxiety that looms around us: what if I don't get better? For all my belief in myself, in my body—I've always recovered from a bad flare-up—that fear hangs over me.

"Tell me I'll be OK," I whisper to Bill as he runs his palms down the back of my head and spine at night.

"You'll get better, you'll get better." His breath is warm against my neck, his voice agitated and impatient.

I need these incantations, the force of repetition, these words that speak of a world righting itself, a body that can be reassembled.

I'm still in bed in mid-November when Lisa stations herself cross-legged on my quilt to help me choose a couple of shirts for Bill's birthday, "L.L.Bean" and "The Territory Ahead" catalogues spread before her. She's mothering me, taking on that encouraging air people assume around the ill, her eyes generous and edgy. A yarn-dyed, true blue dobby shirt? A dark amber, crosshatched cotton corduroy? I'm exhausted from our brief consultation, pointing to pictures, gesturing.

This is where we all three gather, among my tangled blankets and snaking cord of the electric heating pad, when a few weeks later Bill tears open the package Lisa has wrapped. We three on the bed in uneasy intimacy. I can see the strain in their faces. Bill gives me a tense hug, Lisa burbles something cheerful, glancing between us to see if we're OK. Ten minutes, birthday over.

In early December, I prop myself against pillows in a determined attempt to read a client manuscript—they're piling up on my desk. Just ten pages, I tell myself. But the words take on a wavy, distorting sheen I can't absorb, as if my eyes won't connect to my brain. It's like trying to read in some drug-induced haze. I can't do it. Bill has been returning calls from my clients. "Tell them I'll be back in the office after the holidays," I whisper weakly. I'll be able to work by January, I'm sure.

Bill moves around in a gloom, spends long hours in the kitchen skinning chicken and potatoes. He doesn't understand this person of incessant needs who has replaced the woman he fell in love with, or what fate has delivered him to this job of parent to ravenous infant. Evenings, he carries a tray of dinner for himself into our dim bedroom and pulls up the lounge chair next to the bed. This man who feeds me six times a day sits down, tired, to feed himself. He watches the news. I watch him eat, balancing the bamboo tray on his knees. Silhouetted in the pulsing light of the TV and the waning day, his familiar, boyish profile is stoically remote. In his early fifties, Bill is one of those men who still has his chinline, his waistline, and all his wavy brown hair. He's a small man, a runner, with the tight physique and easy stride of a jock.

I'll never forget his compact body in silver-gray nylon running shorts coming at me on the Strawberry Canyon firetrail some eight years ago, the day after we first made love, and the sheer delight that spread over his face when he recognized me. I'd left his place late the night before. To see each other like this in shorts and stark sunlight seemed teasingly illicit.

We shuffled around for a few scintillating moments. I was just heading out down the eucalyptus-studded trail that runs behind the U.C. Berkeley space sciences lab and through the dry hills. He was returning. A dusty heat rose from the ground, the hot earth smell mulched with a musty underlayer of blackberry vines and shade.

"You come here, too?" He seemed pleased that we had this in common. "Working for Peace and Development" read his black T-shirt under a colorful graphic of African women balancing baskets on their heads.

The midday sun drenched us. He cocked his head. For a charged, teetering instant he seemed to be weighing whether to turn back and join me down the path, then he tossed an impish grin over his shoulder and jogged on up the hill to the parking lot.

He hasn't run in weeks. In bed, though we settle automatically, back to stomach, his arm flung over my breast, the distance between us is palpable. I can't talk. Can't write notes in the dark. So much remains unspoken. In these moments what I miss most are our late night conversations against the comfort of each other's body, when words filled the dark—bits and pieces of politics, news, remembered jokes, something we'd heard on the radio—winding out in that careless, end-of-the-day way. Sometimes I'd mumble—I'm more the talker than Bill—and he wouldn't catch what I was saying or I could tell he was falling off, but it wouldn't matter. These conversations were like our daily walks, something to pick up again the next day. It's as if one of us has left, this halt in our exchange.

"I dwell alone, I dwell alone, alone." Rossetti's lament has stayed with me. I believe she meant an aloneness of spirit, an irrevocable sense of being unjoined, whether to another, to her God, or to a world that fit her sensibilities. I'm beginning to understand how layered loneliness is, how built up, like accumulated grime, of individual moments and small acts of misunderstanding and disconnection. But if pain arose from Rossetti's aloneness, so did a reservoir of self, something vibrant, vocal, in fact, irrepressible. "Good poems," poet Richard Wilbur has said, "release us from inarticulateness, which is a great misery." Her poems sprang from her aloneness, a place teeming with language and noise.

4

That Name

The word "fatigue" is such a misnomer for what I was experiencing. I
basically felt like I was dying.
    —Kim Snyder, quoted on *The Infinite Mind*, public radio WNYC

Sometime in 1989 my friend Susan H. handed me a short clipping from the *San Francisco Chronicle*. I have only a vague memory of standing in my yellow-painted entry hall—she must have just
stopped by—as she fished in her purse, waves of russet-blond hair cur-
taining her face, then handed me the newsprint as if she'd almost forgotten. Her words I remember clearly. "I'll bet this is what you've had."

I unfolded the column of print and held it to the light. In matter-of-
fact prose, the article described an illness newly recognized by the
Centers for Disease Control, "chronic fatigue syndrome."

My attention was instantly focused, as if someone had grabbed
me by the shoulders. I read the piece several times, the words coagulat-
ing until a frisson of comprehension slid down the back of my neck.
Chronic fatigue syndrome. Could this be what I'd struggled with since
1980, what I'd called my "recurring virus"? The one no doctor believed
was real?

It was one of those lightbulb moments, those rare revelatory
instants that happen only a few times in life, when disparate, scattered
particles in your brain fly together. In the seventh grade I'd had one
of those moments, when my French teacher, pleased with how easily I
parroted the oral drills, pulled me aside after class and placed a small,

hardbound French book in my hands. A petite, silver-haired man, he held down a remote patch of the schoolyard in an old bungalow, as if foreign languages were always some distant function involving arduous travel, in this case past the leers of the boys in agriculture. I remember the stifling heat of the L.A. afternoon, the relaxed stillness of that bungalow, all the students gone, rows of yellow wooden desks. I was bare-armed in a sundress.

I opened a page, turned several more. I'd never seen written French. Our lessons were completely oral. But as this small man with precise gestures watched, a gleam of pleasure in his eye as if bringing civilization to the outposts, I began reading aloud. My tongue formed the sounds with only a few stumblings, the strange words unloosing their sense. I'll never forget the zing of energy along my nerves as I stood in that empty classroom and felt those odd groups of letters take on sound and meaning, felt the startle of a prior, subtle knowledge brought to the surface.

I stared at the newsprint with that same prickle of astonishment and recognition. I'd always known I had a chronic virus, known the doctors I'd seen throughout the 1980s didn't understand. When I'd asked about Epstein-Barr virus—I must have heard about it in the news—my internist gave an irritated wave of dismissal. "Everyone has antibodies to Epstein-Barr. It's insignificant." Not until 1986, six years into my illness, did I come across a doctor who acknowledged with a shrug that there was such a thing as postviral syndromes. "We don't know much about them," was all he had to say.

Chronic fatigue syndrome. Named and recognized by the CDC. This was a validation, a lining up of things that had been jangled and at odds. "Huh," I said.

Satisfying and juicy as this moment was, it didn't shake my world. It wasn't that I didn't think about it. But by the end of the 1980s my health had significantly improved, and aside from the initial jolt that settled quickly into "of course," this new knowledge was filed away in that place for things I didn't have time to focus on. I was chauffeuring my fifteen-year-old daughter—picture braces and purple eye shadow—to the ACT I movie theater on Shattuck Avenue, following her adamant instructions to drop her off a block away so the boy she was meeting wouldn't see me, after answering for the third time her nervous "Is my hair OK?" and praying I wouldn't have to worry about "you know" for a few more years. And as if adolescent idioms were contagious, I found myself caught up in romance myself. I was racing around the Bay Area to give workshops and classes in fiction writing, where we delved into the intricacies of fictive worlds, then back home for barbecued ribs with my new love, Bill, where I was satisfied with the corporeal and real. Fiction, love, and teenagers, enough distraction. That name, CFS, floated as a shadowy, curious headline to a life in the past, one, thank goodness, I seemed to be leaving behind.

It would be many more years before I learned about the anger and activism this name has spawned. Many more years before I understood the passions generated by a label that doesn't begin to convey the severity of this disease. Pianist Keith Jarrett, who came down with CFIDS in 1997, says, "It's stupid to call it chronic fatigue syndrome. It should be called the forever dead syndrome."[1] And as others have pointed out, defining this disabling illness by the single symptom fatigue is like calling diabetes chronic thirst syndrome or cancer chronic tumor syndrome. It doesn't capture it.

The moment the name was set in print, patients lambasted it as trivializing a serious, debilitating illness and inviting psychiatric stigma. While I was munching on those barbecued ribs with my sweetie, blissfully unconcerned with the new moniker for my illness, an unseen drama was unfolding around me.

On April 15, 1989, in San Francisco at a national conference about chronic fatigue syndrome, patient advocate Thomas Hennessy, Jr., publicly called for a name change. Ill since the mid-1980s after a career in sales and marketing, Hennessy is not the kind of guy to take things lying down. His Web site and e-mails are full of exhortations, capital letters, and exclamation points. On that day, his exclamatory fervor was directed at the researchers and physicians in the audience. "I said, 'If you do nothing else today, change the goddamn name of this disease. It demeans the people who suffer so badly, it sheds no light on a cause or treatment, it does not differentiate this condition from any other chronic condition, and makes no mention of the tremendous pain, and the completely disabling neurological symptoms that we all experience.' The patients in the audience erupted in applause, and many of the doctors looked mystified. The doctors thought, 'What is the big deal? It's just a name.'"[2]

At an earlier conference in 1988 of patients and support group leaders in Portland, Oregon, Seymour Grufferman, a cancer epidemiologist interested in the virus/cancer link, said, presciently, "You are not going to get a fair shake if you call yourself the Chronic Fatigue Syndrome Association, because that carries with it a judgment. Your group should be renamed as well as the disease."[3] He suggested calling the illness chronic fatigue and immune dysfunction syndrome (CFIDS), in recognition of the immune disorder he believed characterized the illness. It was a minor act of rebellion, a harbinger of what was to come.

The name for this illness, rather like the illness itself, has always been a work in progress. In fact, the first name assigned to it rang with respectability. When the mystery illness began surfacing in the United States in the early 1980s, followed by a cluster in Incline Village, Nevada, in the mid-'80s, a number of researchers and physicians initially suspected the Epstein-Barr virus (EBV) to be playing a role. Though EBV—a member of the herpes family and the virus responsible for mononucleosis—is ubiquitous, and the great majority of the U.S. population shows antibodies to it, some physicians believed there was a correlation between abnormally elevated EBV serologies and the viral-like illness that was dragging patients to their offices.

In April of 1985, the National Institute of Allergy and Infectious Diseases (NIAID) held a consensus conference at which, despite some skepticism, the name "chronic Epstein-Barr virus" (CEBV) was used and, as a result, gained broader circulation.[4] In 1987 a patient group, the CEBV Association (later to become the CFIDS Association of America), was founded by patients Marc Iverson and Alan Goldberg in Charlotte, North Carolina. Prestigious medical journals referred to CEBV as a legitimate disease.

The legitimacy was short-lived. Many within the medical community questioned the link between elevated levels of EBV and the symptoms of the illness, and within a few years, the diagnosis fell into disfavor. In 1988, signaling this shift, investigator Gary Holmes at the CDC and his associates, charged with naming the puzzling illness, came up with the name "chronic fatigue syndrome" and the "Holmes criteria" that defined the illness by a list of major and minor symptoms.[5] Among other names, these investigators considered but dismissed "postviral syndrome," because they didn't have definitive proof of a viral agent, as well as "neuromyasthenia" and "myalgic encephalomyelitis," citing a lack of solid evidence of muscle weakness and brain or spinal cord inflammation, which these names imply.[6] It was one of those seemingly innocuous bureaucratic acts with untold consequences.

This semantic vagrancy had a devastating impact on patients, shifting the illness from one of viral origin, CEBV (read, organic), to an unknown origin, CFS (read, raised eyebrows). Ever since, outraged patients have mounted an unprecedented name-change movement. It's an insurrection that brings wheelchair-bound patients and professional lobbyists to Capitol Hill, and spurs letter-writing campaigns by people so ill they can barely lift a pen. It brings angry demands at scientific conferences and teary declarations of lives devastated by illness, jobs and families lost, disability denied. It creates multiple fissures within the patient community as debates swirl about whether to change the name, and if so, how, and to what? It forces scientists to confront issues at the heart of medical practice: how are diseases defined and named? Who has this power? What are the consequences?

The emotions this illness ignites on all sides signal a monumental struggle over medical authority. CFIDS patients stand as an insistent rebuke to the expertise of researchers and physicians, who regard naming as their turf. Typically, any shift in the name of an illness—hysterical paralysis to multiple sclerosis; consumption to TB; melancholia to depression—happens through the medical literature, as researchers refine their understanding of the disease cause or process. But despite significant and mounting evidence of immunologic, neurologic, and autonomic nervous system dysfunction in CFS, researchers insist we don't yet have a clear enough understanding of the pathophysiology of this illness to justify a name change. When you live life *in extremis,* as those with CFIDS do, the dictums of medical science appear rigid and maddening.

There is no question that diagnostic labels exert a powerful effect on physician and public attitudes toward an illness. A 1999 study of medical trainees by Dr. Leonard Jason of DePaul University is a case in point: trainees responded differently to a case study of a patient with classic symptoms of CFIDS depending on the name given to the patient's condition.[7] Of those who were told the patient had Florence Nightingale disease (FN) or chronic fatigue syndrome (CFS), 42 percent and 41 percent, respectively, believed the patient was likely to get better. Of those told the patient had myalgic encephalopathy (ME—a variant of myalgic encephalomyelitis), only 16 percent believed it likely the patient would improve. The results, say the study's authors, "suggest that medical trainees perceive the ME label as being indicative of a more chronic and debilitating illness as compared to the labels of CFS or FN,"[8] no surprise to CFIDS patients. Bonnie Gorman, RN, with the Massachusetts CFIDS Association, ran into a familiar roadblock when her organization tried to raise funds for medical research on CFIDS. "The medical profession is very resistant to taking this illness seriously because of the name. They can't get past the name."[9]

Advocates are furious that the name-change bar is being held so high, pointing out that other illness names have been changed for compassionate reasons (Mongolian idiot syndrome to Down syndrome, leprosy to Hansen's disease) or with less understanding of the disease than we currently have for CFIDS (gay-related immune deficiency to AIDS). The result, they claim, has always been more funding and research, and greater scientific and public acceptance.

My initial blasé attitude toward the name CFS didn't last. In the early 1990s my health began a downward spiral, my office calendar recording the decline by its increasingly large expanse of white, its emptiness. Where there had been three or four writing clients listed each day, there were now two, then one, then only two a week: one client Tuesday at 1:00, one client Thursday at 1:00, the rest of the week blank, an absence that looked like vacation but concealed a struggle.

Something else was happening, too. Muscle aches, like a spreading infection, ran down my limbs. They came in cycles, waxing and waning, seizing me for weeks then lifting. This was new. Earlier I'd joked, parodying those who claim CFIDS is an emotional illness, that my illness was "all in my head": brain fog, sinus pain, sore throat, earache, swollen glands. Ominously, its territory was enlarging. My whole body now registered its distress.

The pungent allure of bay trees and eucalyptus still drew Bill and

me on weekends to our favorite loop of the firetrail behind the U.C.
Berkeley stadium, a path that winds through low hills and canyons,
sweeping between shady inland ridges and wide, sunlit views of the Bay.
When we first met, much of the time I could manage to go a mile and a
half, to a bench that perched on an out-jutting curve like a seat on the
bow of a boat, before turning back. We'd pause for a moment to scan the
Bay's blue-white glitter and watch the ocean fog send its elongated drifts
under the Golden Gate Bridge. We'd tramped far enough to feel we'd
really gone somewhere, gotten away. These walks, our bare legs kicking
up dust, were exhilarating, something we shared. But those hikes were
long gone. Now after half a mile I'd find a spot to rest amid the rutted
dirt and eucalyptus droppings while Bill continued over those familiar
rises and bends. After a while he'd reappear on the ridge and we'd trudge
together back to the car. I was often too exhausted even for that short
excursion.

My doctor, a compassionate man, shrugged and told me he felt for
me. I undertook an elaborate series of phone calls and referrals to find
a doctor within my HMO who supposedly knew something about
CFIDS—a Herculean effort comparable to penetrating the inner recesses of the KGB. I found myself in a small cubicle with Dr. X. When I
began telling him my health was going downhill he smirked, "Come on.
My *grand*mother is going downhill."

Dismissed from his office, I descended, literally, into the underground corridors of the hospital. In a mad moment of optimism, as if
such a small act could save me, I signed up for a stress reduction class.
The class met in the basement—Western medicine is clear about its
hierarchies. On the first day, fifteen other similarly hopeful souls and I
sat in a circle of metal chairs and revealed what in our life was so overwhelming as to bring us to this early morning meeting in a low-
ceilinged basement room with its heat on the blink. A frosty cold radi-
ated from the floor, a concrete slab covered by a thin utility carpet we

would soon lie down on. The instructor, a fresh-faced young woman with flowing skirt and heartening eyes, inhaled a meditative breath, exuding an aura of calm I couldn't share, focused as I was on the ache building in my muscles and the thought of that floor against my bones.

One woman in a leather jacket had lupus, another, muscled and tough-looking, anxiety. When it was my turn, I said simply that I had chronic fatigue syndrome and needed to build my strength. The woman next to me, her upper torso compacted into a spreading middle, drummed her fingernails metallically on the hollow-tubed chair leg. "Yeah, I'm tired all the time too. I need a nap now when I didn't used to."

Her remark brought a rise of blood to my face. The satisfaction of having a name for this illness had turned shaky, like a romantic attraction gone sour. I was beginning to understand the strained relationship we all had with the label we'd been given.

I gamely tried to say a word or two about this illness being a different animal altogether than ordinary fatigue, like a tornado compared to a summer breeze. I tried to explain the severe weakness and pain, the brain fog and confusion, and that a person seriously ill with CFS can be more debilitated than someone with cancer or heart disease. I got only blank stares, as if I were trying to convince a skeptical jury of my innocence, or perhaps it was my guilt, my status as representative of a biochemical order gone wrong. Clearly, I wasn't convincing.

I drove home that day with a chill, aware of the ironies of trying to find inner serenity in the cold belly of an institution of Western medical knowledge, a monument to the supremacy of technological fixes for what ails us, in a room whose heat doesn't work. I fell into bed, fighting to shore up my spirits. These moments happen, I told myself. They're supposed to become Educational Opportunities. But in fact, this illness requires an enormous and constant faith in oneself, a continual building of inner conviction in the face of the doubters, the ill-informed, the suspicious, the kind and well-meaning. Fortunately, or unfortunately, with the body as daily ally, reporting up its aches and fragilities, conviction is not hard.

   While I took to my bed that fall day in 1993, too stressed and ill to continue the stress reduction class, too exhausted to think further, others, thankfully, were more mobilized. September 1993 was a crucial and nerve-wracking moment for the CFIDS community. A panel of eleven federal scientists had been charged with creating a new case definition for CFS. The definition established by Gary Holmes and associates in 1988 had come under increasing criticism for being overly broad and vague, and for inadvertently selecting patients with psychiatric problems. Advocates were eager for a more targeted definition. But rumor was out that the research community wanted to define the illness by fatigue alone, not by its typical symptoms—cognitive impairment, muscle and joint pain, swollen lymph nodes, sore throat—as was currently the case. Such a move would effectively define the illness out of existence, lumping it with all ambiguous, fatiguing conditions. Because the case definition is used to guide research, diagnose patients, determine issues of disability and direct patient care, the results of this meeting would have a profound effect on the lives of everyone with CFIDS. Patient advocates were up in arms, ready to fight a fatigue-based definition and to demand a name change.

   On September 27, advocates, physicians, researchers, and federal officials converged on Building One, a dark auditorium among the mazelike concrete structures and elevated walkways of the CDC in Atlanta. This is where the emergencies of patients become the plodding business of a bureaucracy. Reading about the public meeting in a bulletin published by the CFIDS Association of America, I get the feeling of contained messiness, like science, or the act of protest itself.[10] It was a carefully controlled and orchestrated encounter—advocates given ten minutes to speak and reminded to confine their comments to the case definition—as if it were possible to corral all the heat and friction generated when science collides with the demands of patients: researchers concerned with scientific credibility, patient groups focused on stigma and misunderstanding.

Also packed into the dim, slope-floored auditorium were representatives from clashing advocacy groups. A number of issues have riddled patient solidarity: whether CFIDS is contagious or not, whether it's attributable to a single pathogen or has multiple causes ("different insult, same result"). But one red-hot dividing line is whether federal officials are seen as clueless, sometimes arrogant bureaucrats, or as conspirators engaged in a deliberate cover-up of a devastating epidemic. The CFIDS Association in North Carolina, a well-funded, mainstream group, though often critical of government officials, attempts to work with them.

Others are deeply suspicious of the federal bureaucracy, among them Thomas Hennessy of RESCIND (Repeal Existing Stereotypes about Chronic Immunological and Neurological Diseases), a self-described "free wheeling, sometimes raucous, group of folks who are not happy with the status quo."[11] RESCIND and the National CFIDS Foundation, a group with offices in Needham, Massachusetts, bristle at the idea that the CFIDS Association adequately represents patient interests. In their publications, words like "liars," "cheats," "biased," "useless" are regularly lobbed at the CFIDS Association, its president and CEO Kim Kenney, and the CDC, all seen as complicit with federal foot-dragging and deceit.

In this charged atmosphere, federal officials took their chairs along a table below the stage—graphically illustrating who has a place at the table. Patient advocates filed into the rows of auditorium seats facing them. The moment she settled into the fifth row, Kim Kenney knew this meeting was headed for disaster. The various patient groups had brought their arsenals: independent researchers to present evidence of immune dysfunction in CFIDS patients; patients to tell their personal stories of CFIDS's devastation. When I speak with Ms. Kenney by phone years later as I piece together the trail of action, the name-change story, her voice still sparks with indignation. "The feds could not have been less interested."[12]

When it was her turn to address the gathering, Ms. Kenney outlined a ten-point plan. She urged the government representatives to amend the case definition to "more accurately describe the symptom complex as one which is a multi-systemic disorder of the entire body, not just chronic fatigue." Along with Marya Grambs, Director of the CFIDS Foundation in San Francisco, and immunologist Nancy Klimas from the University of Miami Medical School, Ms. Kenney also argued for changing the name from chronic fatigue syndrome to chronic fatigue and immune dysfunction syndrome "as an interim step until a definitive marker or an etiologic agent is found."[13]

The government officials weren't buying it, and other advocates weren't buying it either. Tom Hennessy, along with Canadian clinician Byron Hyde of the Nightingale Foundation,[14] was adamant that keeping the word fatigue in the name trivialized the disease and demeaned those who suffer from it. Dr. Hyde, who had earlier excoriated the panel for not including in their ranks clinicians who actually treat CFS patients, insisted, ". . . the whole concept of fatigue has warped our understanding of this illness."[15]

Internist Charles Lapp, representing the Cheney Clinic in Charlotte, North Carolina, agreed: "Fatigue is a given. All of the patients have fatigue. But it's not the fatigue that brings them to my practice for help. . . . It's the cognitive symptoms that are really the most debilitating."[16]

A lineup of patients and clinicians took the mike to offer suggestions for a new name: acquired immunoneurological syndrome (AINS);

AIDS-HIV negative; Gilliam's disease, after Dr. A. G. Gilliam, the assistant surgeon general who described a similar disease in 1938.

No agreement on a name. No support from the federal officials. Patient advocates were even more outraged when they saw a draft of a booklet the officials were circulating entitled "The Facts about Chronic Fatigue Syndrome," which repeated the federal scientists' claim that they had found no clinically significant immune changes in people with CFS. The booklet dismissed studies conducted by anyone other than the CDC, and grossly underestimated the prevalence of CFS, claiming about three to ten thousand people in the United States had the illness, a number that incensed activists. Says Ms. Kenney, "Nearly every statement in the book was a real offense to the patient community."

As government officials continued to insist that you could pull anyone off the street and they would have the same immunologic profile as a CFS patient, "I just sort of lost it," Ms. Kenney recalls.

"How in the world can you say that?" She grabbed the microphone in the aisle.

Chief of the CDC's Viral Exanthems and Herpesvirus Branch, Dr. William Reeves, bald except for a fringe of white hair and a trim white line of beard around his jaw, was impassive. "Well, statistically, that's accurate."

"It just went to hell from there," says Ms. Kenney. "Clearly their intent was to dismiss the immunology. There were four of us from the association at that meeting, and it was the most discouraged any of us had ever been."

Pictures taken on a second day of meetings show the FDA representative doing her nails and a line of federal officials seated at a skirted table, looking as if they're half asleep. One advocate was heard to mutter: "This meeting about the case definition is a sham. It was put on to placate the patients. They are going to go back behind closed doors and do whatever they want."[17]

In the end, activist Marya Grambs, angry and disheartened, took the mike to level the retaliatory shot government representatives most fear: "Believe it or not, those of us presenting today are the polite ones and we are the reasonable ones. There are a great many other CFIDS patients out there who are not so polite or reasonable. And believe me, we can get them here."[18]

In 1994, the CDC issued its revised case definition for CFS, called the Fukuda et al. criteria.[19] To no one's surprise, they did not include a name change, though the official paper did acknowledge the inadequacy of the name "chronic fatigue syndrome." Tempers in the CFIDS community were reaching a boil. When CFS was first named in 1988, many patients had thought both an understanding of the illness and a name change were around the corner. Without these victories, the various factions of the patient community seemed like pinballs careening in every direction.

One group contacted Senator Edward Kennedy's office to convince him to get Congress to mandate a name change. They were told that isn't what Congress does. Fed up with the bureaucracy, many patients simply referred to their illness as myalgic encephalomyelitis (ME), whether the powers-that-be sanctioned that name or not. Convinced by Tom Hennessy of the urgency of the name-change issue, patient Roger Burns, who maintains an informational Web site on CFS, began including editorials on his site and organizing name-change forums at medical meetings.[20]

A number of advocates appealed directly to scientists, regaling them with stories of patients demeaned and dismissed, arguing the urgent need for a name change, to no avail. Many were working with patient groups in Europe, Canada, Australia, and New Zealand and attending international CFS/ME meetings, where they hit another snag: Though the name ME is used in Great Britain, Canada, and other European countries, the definitions for CFS and ME differ. ME advocates in Britain, fighting their own battle for legitimacy, were adamant that CFS patients in the United States not adopt the name ME, fearing this move would undo their effort to distinguish between the neurocognitive illness ME and the more inclusive, fatigue-based definition of CFS.

The leadership of the CFIDS Association was grappling with its own questions. Though the Association always acknowledged the importance of a name change, many in the organization felt too much focus on this issue could siphon energy from other concerns: public awareness, the research effort, expanding federal funding for CFIDS. They were starting to hear from members who felt the name issue wasn't as important as some were making it out to be, that there were more significant things to focus on. "Until science gives us a clear name, don't spin your wheels on that."

The improvisational dance stuttered forward. The National CFIDS Foundation and RESCIND, along with many patients, accused the CFIDS Association of not pursuing the name change vigorously enough. The CFIDS Association cranked out fact sheets listing all their efforts. Disgruntled advocates cried, "Liars! Cheats!"

Patient advocacy movements have always been fluid and diffuse, but the reality was hitting. From the cloak-and-dagger conspiracy theorists of the National CFIDS Foundation to the more moderate CFIDS Association to the isolated patient struggling to work and pay the bills— what was the prospect of such a disparate coalition of people, most of whom were seriously ill, mounting a successful campaign to change the name of an affliction with no known cause, in the face of opposition from the scientific community?

5

The Erotics of Illness

... illness often takes on the disguise of love, and plays the same odd tricks.

—Virginia Woolf, "On Being Ill"

December 1995

Pale early winter light streaks our room. Bill hunches into the curved-beechwood chair next to our bed, elbows on knees. He's been for a run along the Strawberry Canyon firetrail, breathing the largeness of open space. He needs to get out, now that I'm always in. In bed. All day, all night. He needs those hills and trails, that influx of oxygen. He bows his head so I can see only the ridge of his brow, then the air seems to go out of him. He raises his eyes to me, haggard.

"You need to see a therapist."

Every raw nerve in my body fires with electrifying force. I shoot up from bed, knifing the air with my palms.

This is a caustic, stinging affront. Proof that he doesn't understand me, doesn't understand this illness. Proof of how alone I am. That even my most intimate relationship, what should be a bastion of understanding and care, is contaminated by the dismissal and disbelief of the culture is the ultimate blow.

I snatch a sheet of paper from my bedside table and scrawl huge, angry words. "You have no idea what you're saying. I'm too weak, too ill! I can't talk! I just need to rest."

We fight, a comic implosion, like a silent movie. I scribble furious notes and Bill paces with a tensile agitation in the narrow corridor between our bed and the microwave, voice low, since he knows yelling will hurt my ears. "You can't see yourself the way I can, your anxiety, your fears."

We lob fragmented accusations—the kind we'll cringe at later, or deny, or rewrite, "No, you . . ."—hurling them with all the percussive force we can muster in silence. There is something huge in us that neither of us can get out. I slump back on the pillow, waves of exhaustion weighing me.

Bill goes to the window and stares, arms crossed, his body rigid against contained emotion. He seems lost somewhere between anger and hopelessness. My illness breathes as a palpable presence in the room. I imagine it runs through his body as a nightmare of responsibility and dependence, his, mine. There are many perversities to this illness—to any illness—and this is one of them: it has come between us as a painful wedge at the same time that it has thrown us together in a steamy, flailing intimacy. We're both trying to figure out what's going on. This person I've lived with for eight years—now frightened, wary—is suddenly new. I don't know him. Sprawled in bed, stringy haired, I'm not the person he thought he knew either.

A "new marriage," English critic John Bayley calls it, euphemistically, this quagmire of illness and love. In *Elegy for Iris*, Bayley writes eloquently of how he watched his wife Iris Murdoch slip into the darkness of Alzheimer's. He describes their shifting relationship, this new marriage, as one of increased closeness and merging, altering that "happy apartness which marriage had once taken wholly for granted."[1] Ours feels more like an old marriage to me, pummeled and frayed. Fusion become abrasive and claustrophobic.

Illness and love are disturbingly linked. Maybe this is what is so frightening about both states—the intense vulnerability, the way mundane life disappears, the specter of dependency and disruption, the all-consuming, chaotic reality that overtakes you. Ordinary work comes to a halt. Phone calls aren't returned, floors aren't mopped. You're in bed, immersed in the needs of the body. But ours has become a one-directional affair. Bill is worn out, tired of tending to my needs. I'm too much for him.

I flick on my Sony Walkman and stick the tiny plastic knobs in my ears. Harps, flutes, strings. The lilting, soothing music of eagles soaring on mountain updrafts, of expansive skies and cumulus clouds, a harmony I plug into my body. Downstairs, the kitchen is a splotchy clutter of milk-filmed bowls, burnt juices encrusting grimy pie tins, stacked saucepans. Crumbs of cauliflower, oatmeal flakes, and decomposing things fleck the floor. All around me are wadded, tea-stained napkins and soggy plates. Illness is nothing if not inelegant.

Bill leaves for a meeting. In the late afternoon I squirm my way over to our bedside chair as the sun sets. I've always reveled in this transitional, twilight moment when the world seems infinitely vibrant, opening its underlayer of color. The slanted sun throws a salmon tint on our white bedroom walls. Outside, the neighbor's towering Chinese elm, color-engorged, bursts with glossy emerald light.

But tonight I watch the dusk with growing apprehension. I'm fading, in need of dinner, my brain thickening in its mossy confusion. Bill is late coming home. The broad limbs of spiked Monterey pine needles outside my window darken to black clumps against a pale sky. A window across the way lights an orange square behind the branches.

The white-lidded cooler glints next to me, empty. Five o'clock, no Bill. I eye the clock like a buzzard. Five fifteen. I scavenge the cooler for leftover bites of toast, three final slivers of canned peach. I can last another fifteen minutes. As if hypoglycemic, I become light-headed and shaky when hunger strikes. A foggy disorientation envelopes me. My aches magnify, the pressure that bores through my head down my spine mounts, as if someone has packed my bones with lead.

As the room falls into darkness, I'm infused with that potent mix of anger and frustration at my helpless state, at being left. My brain weighs my growing weakness against my faith in Bill's imminent return. I rehearse in my mind how I might pull myself up, navigate the mountainous stairs, cross the open plains of the dining room, reach the remote regions of the kitchen. Just as I hit a point of dazed determination and hoist myself up, I hear the familiar snug scrape of the front door. Tottering at the top of the stairs, I meet Bill with mute, pained exhaustion. Without a word, he pivots to the kitchen to crack an egg in the frying pan.

He goes for two days without looking at me or talking other than terse, mechanical questions. Do you want more soup? Potatoes or rice? His face is pinched, body steeled against feeling. What runs through my head as I watch him—besides the seething torrent of words I have to dam up inside, that I can't let out—is that he looks as exhausted as I do. He appears emptied out, that kind of fatigue where you have to shield your eyes from light, where everything is too much to take in.

On our second date—the first having been a walk out the Tilden Park trail to Inspiration Point, as if we were going to need inspiring—I swooned through dinner at a Cambodian place, from fatigue, not infatuation, and begged off the second set at Yoshi's, a local jazz club where I'd barely been able to mumble a few coherent sentences to the friends of Bill's we'd gone to meet. Dating in a state of exhaustion—this was 1987; I didn't yet know there was such a thing as CFIDS—is an exercise in self-impersonation. I could usually pull things off during the day. Evenings were touch-and-go.

Despite the inauspicious beginnings, we tried again the next weekend. There was something about his impassioned defense, waving his fork in the air, of his unsweetened blintzes that piqued my interest. He told the story of how his Protestant mother labored for years to re-create his Jewish father's exact memory of *his* mother's sugarless blintzes.

When Bill worked as breakfast cook at David Rosenthal's delicatessen during law school, he'd refused to sweeten the hundreds of blintzes he rolled and filled each week. "I told David my father would kill me if I put sugar in them!" A zealous cook, a plaintiff's lawyer, and a former political scientist who could give a good riff on Third World development policy and democratization in Nicaragua and El Salvador. This was interesting.

When Bill suggested dinner again, I was ready to rest all week and patch myself together for a similar act. Instead he blurted, "You know, I usually go to bed early."

"Oh, me too!" I cried, and we happily unloaded our brief charades as nightlife aficionados, for which, thankfully, Bill had much less tolerance than I. I was guiltily relieved to discover Bill had some kind of recurring "episode," as he called it, that left him achy and fatigued, especially after a cold or flu, for months at a time. If he tried to run during these episodes, he'd be exhausted for days or weeks afterward. Fatigue, exercise intolerance, flare-ups after colds. We had an unsought bond, though at the time it seemed more nebulous, less immediate than the spirited debates we had about Catherine MacKinnon and the politics of pornography, or the pleasure we found in each other, always early.

We've all heard stories of couples who take on parallel afflictions. One gets arthritis, the other's back goes out. In line with this empathic tradition, Bill's lingering malaise, after having gotten better in recent years, is back. Allergies? Depression? His own viral onslaught, worn adrenals, caretaker's exhaustion, who knows? We often wondered if Bill had some version of CFIDS. And we wondered how careful we needed to be about my illness. Was I contagious? Did we need to take precautions? Were we passing something back and forth? Physicians had no answers. Most lacked basic information about the illness itself, let alone about the risk of transmission or need for precautions. But as I survey my romantic history, the picture is disturbing.

Only in retrospect do the details assume significance. Summer 1980. I'm standing with a lover in the small foyer of my second-story flat on Claremont Avenue in Oakland. Victorian flowered wallpaper and dark walnut trim. We've just gotten up from bed; he's about to leave for a meeting. I'm jazzed, in love with this balding man with the trim, professorial beard and brown eyes that penetrate mine. And I'm swimming with fatigue and brain fog. Just a couple months earlier I'd come down with that nasty virus that wasn't going away.

When I sag against the wall and hold my head, a knowing look crosses his face. He touches his fingers to his temples with that sly, vaudevillian smile he had. "You get that too? Feeling like your brain is made of cottage cheese?" I think of this many years later. He knew those symptoms. He worked himself ragged, was often worn and dragging. Was it just overwork? Or did he also have this illness? Did I give it to him? Did he give it to me?

A year and a half earlier I'd been hit with a vicious case of mononucleosis, caught from another man I was dating. Blond, full-bearded, vigorous, he'd come to the bookstore where we both worked pale-faced and exhausted. I thought he'd had the flu. It never occurred to me to think I shouldn't kiss him. Such innocent days. Then there were the luscious hours spent in a green VW bug parked at Santa Monica beach when I was seventeen, from which I emerged with a magnificent crush and a fat herpes blister on my mouth, and the fact that at least one study has shown people with CFIDS to have higher antibody levels to herpes 1 and 2 than the general population.[2] Am I paying for my past? Are we all?

These moments of infection all shimmer in my mind as tender and memorable. Silently brewing with future malaise. The gray-white patches, mottled like chicken membrane, that line my throat, the swollen nodes under my jawbone, are the visible markings of a past still lodged in my body. This is the lesson of contagion, that we live in an invisible web of interconnectedness, never knowing which strand will loop through our own body, alter our cells. We're all having relationships we don't know about with people we've never met, interconnected by microbial travel, invisible lanes of traffic, our bodies the superhighways. What these delightful moments of microbial transfer say about my choice of boyfriends is clear. What they say about CFIDS, though, is more complicated.

The issue of contagion doesn't get talked about much anymore, but for a while in the 1980s and '90s, it was a contentious, hot-button issue. Citing illness clusters, multiple cases within families, and an infectious onset, many people became frightened that they were seeing an infectious epidemic. The contagion claim was about fear, about wanting federal officials to take this illness seriously, and above all about belief, each person putting forth the adamantly held origin story for his or her brain fog and exhaustion: It was the upper respiratory infection I caught from my boyfriend. It was the mononucleosis I never recovered from.

Most physicians and scientists dismissed the idea of contagion. And sparring with those who insisted CFS was contagious was a vocal contingent of persons with CFIDS (PWCs) who were convinced they had a compromised immune system, most likely environmentally induced, first and foremost. They advanced an equally adamant origin story: It was the chemicals at the photo lab where I worked. It's the toxins in our homes, our land, our air, disrupting our immune and neuroendocrine systems. These two camps, virus versus immune dysregulation, were reviving the old "seed or soil" debate that in the late 1880s set Louis Pasteur against his colleague Claude Bernard. Pasteur, of course, championed the microbe's role in disease. Bernard advanced the argument that the terrain of the illness, the internal environment of the body, contributed as much to illness as the invading pathogen.[3] (When he suffered a stroke and was treated with leeches behind the ears, even Pasteur had to acknowledge the microbe wasn't everything.)

If a virus or other infectious agent is involved in CFIDS, is it the cause of the illness, or is it secondary to an immune disorder that allows previously latent viruses, such as herpes simplex or EBV or HHV-6, to reemerge? Are the symptoms of CFIDS the result of a chronic viral infection that the immune system can't control, or a onetime infection that initiates chronic overactivation of the immune system, or a reactivation of formerly latent pathogens in immune-compromised individuals? Despite the latest incarnation of the legendary Pasteur/Bernard dispute, today most would agree the seed or soil fight is rooted in a simplistic dichotomy. But following the fissures of the contagion debate, like tracing cracks in a dry riverbed, reveals the evolution and complexity of thinking about CFIDS itself.

In the mid- and late 1980s, a number of patient activists and some clinicians who treated the emerging disease speculated that they were seeing an infectious epidemic. Internist Dan Peterson, who treated patients in the Incline Village, Nevada, outbreak in 1985, claimed there was "*some* contagion by *some* route," though that route—blood? saliva? sexual activity? through the air?—was unclear.[4] Yet most physicians and researchers, who were skeptical of the disease to begin with, rejected the idea of an infectious illness.

In 1992, when Dr. Anthony Komaroff and his colleagues published their study of the 1985 Nevada outbreak in the *Annals of Internal Medicine,* they cautiously noted the possibility of an infectious origin. "Enough cases occurred among family members, co-workers, and other close contacts to suggest the possibility of an infectious agent transmissible by casual contact."[5] Tahoe wasn't the only cluster outbreak. Among others, there was an outbreak within an orchestra in Raleigh, North Carolina, in August of 1984, and among residents of the working-class desert town Yerington, Nevada, in 1985. Over one hundred adults and children in Lyndonville, New York, became ill in 1985–86. In his 1990 study of seventy-four children with CFIDS in Lyndonville, Dr. David

Bell found that almost 64 percent had another family member with the illness.[6]

I myself was in the midst of a Bay Area cluster when, throughout the 1980s, I limped through my day in a fugue state of exhaustion, believing I was just a run-down single parent—a fact that hints at the many undiagnosed, unrecognized cases of CFIDS. Unbeknownst to me, in 1989 internist Carol Jessop was seeing over 1,100 patients with an illness similar to mine in her East Bay practice.[7] Of course clusters don't prove contagion—clusters of CFIDS within families can indicate genetic factors, and within families or communities could be due to noninfectious environmental exposures (chemicals, toxins).[8] But some activists continued to raise red flags. A 1991 informal surveillance study showed that 10 to 15 percent of patients with CFIDS had another household member suffering from the disease.[9] Interestingly, the National Institutes of Health (NIH) and the Centers for Disease Control (CDC) each studied the illness within its infectious disease division.

The debate boiled over in 1996 with the publication of Hillary Johnson's *Osler's Web: Inside the Labyrinth of the Chronic Fatigue Syndrome Epidemic.* In March of that year, promoting her book on *Good Morning America* and *Prime Time Live,* Ms. Johnson pronounced CFIDS to be a "very contagious brain disease." In the ensuing uproar, even Dr. Anthony Komaroff asserted that "There's no proof that CFS is contagious," and most physicians and federal investigators concurred.[10] Virologist Jay Levy of the University of California, San Francisco, who had investigated a viral agent in CFS, stated flatly, "CFIDS is not a contagious disease. . . . The illness represents a hyperactive immune response, most likely to common infectious agents, particularly viruses, that do not give long-term harmful effects to most people. The onset of CFIDS is determined by a person's own genetic make-up and not by a contagious agent."[11]

Patients, too, were wary of Ms. Johnson's definitive claim. She provided an invaluable service to those with CFIDS by proclaiming on a national stage that CFIDS was a serious and devastating illness and by exposing in detail the federal government's failure to respond to a growing public health crisis. Many PWCs hailed her book as a vital and groundbreaking investigation. Yet her unequivocal claim of contagion worried many others who feared stigma and rejection by those around them. "If you think we were isolated yesterday," wrote one woman, "how will we be treated tomorrow? Contagion hasn't been proven! Hillary Johnson is doing us more harm than good."[12]

Today the consensus is that there is no clear evidence that CFIDS is contagious, certainly not casually contagious. We'd be seeing different epidemiological patterns if it were. Though there's some evidence CFIDS may be linked to an unresolved or persistent infection, to date, no single infectious agent has been shown to be responsible for CFIDS. It's possible that CFIDS is caused by a still unidentified virus, or co-infection with two or more pathogens. But the role of inciting or opportunistic infections and the possible impact of an altered immune system remain to be elucidated. The bottom line, as always, is that much more research is needed.

It seems clear that a complex illness like CFIDS (one publication referred to it as "one of the most fascinating and complex maladies of modern medicine"![13]) isn't going to be understood with the old one-pathogen-one-disease model. An interactive network, like an intricate electrical grid, of instigating and perpetuating factors is more likely. What does this mean exactly? I put in a phone call to Dr. Bell in his office in Lyndonville, New York, where he still sees CFS patients. After two decades of hands-on work treating and studying CFS, he has come to see this illness as a postinfectious dysautonomia (autonomic nervous system dysfunction). "What that means," he says, "is that an infection initiates a process whereby the immune system starts overreacting. And that process then causes reduction in cerebral blood flow, abnormalities in the HPA axis [a key part of the endocrine system], and a variety of other things."[14]

Complicated indeed: an immune system that is overreacting, reduced blood flow to the brain, defects in the autonomic system, which controls heart beat and blood pressure, abnormalities in the endocrine system, which regulates production of hormones. Adding to the complexity, the disease process may not be the same in all people with CFIDS. Just as a painful, swollen joint can be caused by infection, injury, or arthritis, the symptoms of CFIDS may be the end result of different processes in different people.

Dr. Bell is an amiable man who seems pleased to expand on his ideas. His voice rises with enthusiasm when he describes several recent studies that have created quite a buzz. "One is the Dubbo study by the CDC. Extraordinary study. Wonderful science. What they're doing is, in the county of Dubbo, Australia, they're prospectively looking at all cases of Epstein-Barr virus, Ross River virus, and Q fever, illnesses known to sometimes have a chronic aftermath. And they are now seeing that 10 percent of these people go on to develop chronic fatigue syndrome. . . . This is implying that those three infections cause CFS in otherwise healthy people. That's very interesting.

"The other study . . . that just knocked my socks off was hepatitis C. This was a study done by a hepatitis specialist who was treating hepatitis C with interferon [a protein that is part of the body's antiviral response]. . . . Seventy percent developed marked fatigue, and 30 percent developed chronic fatigue syndrome. So it was the interferon treatment that caused the CFS, not the actual virus circulating in their system. . . . The CFS is the immune response from infection."[15] This finding is consistent with the idea that the symptoms of CFS could be precipitated by an immune system in overdrive.

Some researchers have been focusing on twin studies to investigate the role of genetics in CFIDS. In phase I of a study of twins at the

University of Washington, Dedra Buchwald and associates turned up evidence that hints at a genetic component. Studying 146 female twin pairs in which one twin had CFIDS, they found that 55 percent of identical twins both had CFIDS, while only 19 percent of fraternal (nonidentical) twins did.[16] The Dubbo, hepatitis C, and twin studies, along with many others, present an intriguing view of several pieces of the CFIDS puzzle: pathogens, immune overactivation, and genetics.

So back to my Claremont Avenue apartment in 1980, my professorial, brown-eyed lover. His sensuous intensity apparently masked a devastating microbial transfer, one that in another person would have resulted in a onetime infection that cleared up normally, but in a susceptible individual could initiate CFIDS. By all accounts, I was susceptible, having never fully recovered from mononucleosis, rundown from divorce, graduate school, and single parenting, perhaps genetically predisposed. It's possible the mono I'd had a year and a half earlier was the actual initiating event, setting the stage for the next vicious virus that came along to deliver the final punch. Whatever the combination of factors, for me, this lover was a microbial conduit with devastating consequences. Our voluptuous salivary exchange either initiated or furthered the cascade of inner disruptions—of the autonomic nervous system, neuroendocrine system, immune system—that constitutes CFIDS. It's possible that he, too, had some CFIDS-like symptoms for a time, and that he, too, was in some way susceptible. I don't know. That was a long time ago.

The New Year comes, cold and hazily sunny, and with it some relief. The sinus infection that made my head swell up like wet wood finally subsides. I toss out my decongestant, Sudafed, and immediately start sleeping through the night. Propped in my bedside chair, I can even read a client manuscript for half an hour a day, an accomplishment that fills me with elation, muted as it is by the thick pull of gravity on every muscle.

One afternoon I bundle in sweats, a gray hooded sweatshirt tight around my face, and make my way stiffly downstairs. Bill and his friend Paul, watching football, gawk, burritos midair, as if I were an apparition. I feel like one, staring out from my cowl silently. I give a wan smile, step to the front porch, and gaze down the driveway. Pride, joy, sadness—a mix of feelings rakes through me, that the view of a driveway, that coarse, stained cement, crumbling at the edge, weeds in the cracks, should be a thing of celebration. This is the odd consolation and reward for those interminable, sequestered months: a drug-free high in which a strip of concrete is cause for amazement. I pull into my lungs a deep breath of damp winter air.

My world slowly enlarges to a daily venture up the street, one house, then two, but I still inhabit the spaces of recovery, bed, home, garden. I'm still limp with heat and exhaustion, my brain so foggy that every-thing seems out-of-focus. I look out on the neighborhood as if behind a veil, doubly removed from the world.

Bill arrives home one evening with a video tucked under his arm and a hopeful shrug. An offering of sorts, a stab at normalcy. It takes us three nights to get through the movie. Trying to absorb the action, the throbbing light, shifting scenes, even for a short time, exhausts me. But we manage to do it. *Eat, Drink, Man, Woman* is one of those uplifting, reassuring stories, about an Asian family torn by generational conflicts, drawn together by food. Teenage daughters disappear, come home preg-nant, fight, but the father always shuffles in and lays the table with win-ter melon blossom soup, shrimp balls, five spice beef, and sauteed gin-ger duck. They all come back, this fractured family, drawn by some migratory magnet to food, to home. This unremarkable dinner-table moment seems remarkable to me. The simplicity and hopefulness of it all. The power and attraction of that table spread with duck meat and dumplings.

Under the covers, Bill and I stretch along the warmth of each other's body, our uncertainties and tensions momentarily in the background. They're passing the spicy beef, plucking up morsels of onion and sauteed duck, juicy, sizzling, steamy, aromatic. I want all of it, the tangy flavors on my tongue, the long-suffering but forgiving looks, the jostling elbows. I want this meal that can straddle and survive conflict and grief. Watching others feast, the suppressed pain of these last months wells up in me. I twist in bed to grab a tissue and mop my eyes.

Bill, too, is moved. He reaches his arms around my shoulder, a hug of genuine warmth without the weight of despair.

I pull my head back to hold his gaze, inches away. The translucent blue of his eyes always startles me, a thin transparency of color crystalline in its clarity. "I want my life back."

There follows a series of clumsy negotiations as we attempt some semblance of lovemaking. No. My shoulder hurts. Ow. Gentle as Bill is, his fingers register on every sore muscle fiber. The exertion is exhausting; I have to stop several times to catch my breath, my heart racing. Bill is patient. Then a grinning, triumphant amazement at the body's capacity for existing in a polymorphous state of pain and pleasure. For a brief time, the heaviness of my body seems to lift, the pain recede. Those endorphins are truly opiates.

These are stolen moments, proof that what is between us is stronger than the intruder in our lives. Love has become thievery, snatching a clandestine interlude from the real scoundrel and thief, illness. Tomorrow I'll feel battered, overcome with a throbbing fatigue, a bruised pain in the bony ridges of clavicle, shoulder, ribs, as if my tendons and bones are soft and crushable. For now, I run my fingertips down the narrow channel of Bill's spine to the hollow just below his hips, a classic curve smooth as the inside of a conch, and wonder how many more food videos we can get hold of.

"How about cooking shows?" Bill peers at me over the pages of the TV guide. To my relief, most days now I can manage a half-hour of TV as long as it's quiet. Cooking shows are perfect, static pictures broken only by the flick of a wrist or plop of diced onion, calm enough not to fluster my brain. This is progress, from staring into a pot of steaming water to staring at a pot of spaghetti. I love these shows. They take me to another world, where thoughts of pain give way to fascination with a boiling crock of clams—I don't even like clams—or the floury slap of dough. I'm mesmerized by these images, absorbing every bubbling slosh of red pasta sauce, every flake of minced parsley. I lose myself in them, a strange thought, since I want only to gain myself back.

We discover that the public library stocks travel and nature videos. Lisa swings by on her way home from work and brings me a stack, brief moments of escape. Boating down the Danube, tracking orangutans in Borneo, anywhere but here. Among the selections one week I'm thrilled to find a small gem, a twenty-minute short of a woman in her bakery—surrounded by marzipan, buttery icing, glossy strawberry tarts—culminating with her fluid assembly of a three-tiered chocolate wedding cake. I can't get enough of it. Over and over I study the mixer blades paddling thick waves of creamy dark batter, the flat cakes steaming on puckered waxed paper. Then the lather of whipped cream, chocolate disappearing under a drape of white, and the steady absorption that leaves the woman's face intent and peaceful. Her moving fingers. A planting of blue pansies.

In the stripped-down place of illness that allows nourishment but no richness, survival but no extravagance, something in me craves effusion and sensuality, lavish excess. My dreams are filled with full-color food panoramas. Sugar-dusted éclairs. Opulent banquets, the platters of stacked drumsticks, oranges, and apples gleaming in rich ambers and reds.

She likes most of all, the baker says in her calm voice, working alone in the hours before her husband comes in to load his station wagon with afternoon deliveries and their boys race around begging for after-school brownies. I keep staring at this woman alone in her sumptuous sanctuary, gritty sugar coating her fingers, with what can only be described as longing, the kind of rapt attention of a child pressing her nose to the window of a bakery. I imagine her engulfed in chocolaty hot oven air, and all that lusciousness and pleasure emerging from her smooth orchestration.

"Way to go, Mom," Lisa cheers from the doorway as she shuttles in with a bowl of chicken noodle soup.

6

Staying Home

We have to designate the space of our immobility by making it the
space of our being.

—Gaston Bachelard, *The Poetics of Space*

February 1996

I make it to the sidewalk and three houses up the block, marking
these steps the way shot putters mark fractions of an inch, each
micrometer of territory, each expansion of range, a victory, my heavy
body launched a little farther. I pause for a luxurious moment, soaking
in the brilliant winter light like someone who's been underground. As if
tipsy with light themselves, the cherry trees lining our street have broken into a frothy pink flowering, checkering the air with color and exuberance. It feels like an only-in-California, early intimation of spring,
and all wrong. The air is sharp with cold. I'm bundled in my blue-plaid
wool scarf, the rolled rim of my knitted cap pulled over my ears. I usually feel a vague alarm at this yearly February blossoming, at how quickly rain pummels the petals to the ground, flat as wet tissue. But today
this false spring feels like a recaptured moment, intoxicating and sensu-
al, as if I've teased out of grayness a bud of vivid life.

This afternoon my mother and her husband Otto are trundling up
from Santa Barbara in her gray-blue Buick for my sister Suzanne's fifti-
eth birthday and to see this daughter who has faded to a whispery voice
on the phone. The image of my mother chugging around in that bulky
Buick, heavy with chrome, always strikes me as incongruous, as misleading as the mutinous blossoms. Everything about my mother is light,

floating: her baggy cotton slacks, puff-sleeved cotton blouse, her loose ring of gray-white curls, high girlie voice, nose tipped to the sky, a finger pointing upward as if she's had an illumination.

She calls from Suzanne's to arrange a visit, laughter fuzzing through in the background. "We don't want to tire you. Tell us what's best." Always considerate, accommodating. I don't know what private worries she might entertain; with me she is always upbeat. She's been sending get-well cards that she buys on sale and saves till she needs them, with pictures of bunnies and baskets, and words like "best" and "sweet" and "love" underlined with a dash of her blue ballpoint pen.

The next day I pull on a sweatshirt and make my way down to the living room, where she gives me a fervent but careful hug. Otto, sweet man, is full of Ohs and hugs and Look at yous, rolled out in his Danish accent. Nothing makes more clear that you're ill than the solicitous pats and twitters of friends and family, the one who coos from the doorway or clucks from the bedside, the one who praises your ability to walk in those high-pitched tones as if you'd just learned, a tottering one-year-old—an interchangeable coterie chorusing their affection. I wish they'd talk to me like I'm an adult, but I'm too weak to speak up.

Bill washes mugs and passes around steaming mint tea.

Settled around our small living room, Mom, Otto, and Suzanne chat away. What a wonderful birthday party it had been, how regal Suzanne looked, this from Mom in her admiring voice. "All those presents! She looked like a queen."

"You should have seen her," Otto says. There's a soft charitableness to his face, opened in a smile and crested with thick waves of white hair.

Peacock-bright in a silky magenta and chartreuse running suit, Suzanne slides her eyes to him flirtatiously.

I nod my head, an effort that sloshes my Jell-O-brain and makes me woozy. A heavy pressure weights my chest. I sag into a corner of the couch and let their conversation drift around me.

My family is easy, a wash of voices and animations I don't have to join, undemanding comfort. Talking around me like this, oddly, is the most reassuring thing they can do, a way to include me in their ordinariness, their cheer and parties and news, so I can participate, if from an echoing distance.

Mom flutters up, restless from sitting. We take a short stroll, a couple of houses up the street. She patters on about cherry blossoms and eyes me cagily, affecting a casual air. Mom may seem breezy, but she has the senses of a hawk, spotting her target with acuity and precision.

Back in the driveway she raises an impulsive finger. "Any trouble with your eyes?"

"I do have some problems with focusing and . . ."

"Oh, I'm sure it's fine." Snatching back the negative thought. New Age gurus would love my mother, ambassador of positivity and cheer.

I know she's wondering if I might have multiple sclerosis. I don't, but in fact the two conditions have a lot in common: muscle weakness and impairment, vision problems, brain lesions, disequilibrium, a waxing and waning pattern, fatigue, a suspected autoimmune component, and a multifactorial origin, including genetics, environment, and pathogens (HHV-6 and *chlamydia pneumoniae,* in particular, have been suspected in both MS and CFS). The conditions can appear so similar that the diagnoses are often confused—people diagnosed with MS who really have CFS and vice versa. Dr. Anthony Komaroff, one of the foremost CFIDS researchers, shares a number of patients with Harvard's top multiple sclerosis experts, and has commented on this confusion: "There are some patients . . . where we honestly don't know what they have. They could have chronic fatigue syndrome or could have multiple sclerosis. They're on the borderline between the two illnesses. And some of them have gone definitively in one direction over the course of time, and others have gone the other direction."[1] Interesting too that, like CFIDS, MS was initially thought to be psychogenic and ridiculed as "hysterical paralysis," and that the cause of MS remains unknown.

I wave through the living room window as Mom, Otto, and Suzanne sail off, a perverse reversal, since my mother doesn't like to travel and would prefer to stay home, and I should be the one cruising about. All wrong.

I seem to be always looking through windows, like a specimen behind glass. From my bed I gaze up through domed plastic skylights at fragments of sky and flowering apple branches, already leafed out this February and flaunting white pinwheel blooms. Out the east-facing stretch of windows I watch the throaty red flash of a bullet-fast hummingbird, the shrill fights and leaps of squirrels rattling branches of the gangly Monterey pine. Mourning doves and house sparrows rut through pine needles and decomposing leaves, finding them endlessly lucrative.

It's unsettling to be in an environment so familiar that is at the same time foreign, a world I never expected would be so unrelentingly mine. The thought shudders through me: I'm not where I should be. I'm slipping into my mother's world of flower beds and pots and towels. My mother embraces home as she embraces her five daughters, fiercely. Home is where she wants to be, immersed in the steamy familiarity of her kitchen, baking fragrant loaves of banana-nut bread in her heavy, old-fashioned tins, blackened by decades of use. Or out in her garden, pruning her Cecil Bruner roses with sharp, lively jabs. Home is where she feels most alive, most herself. The walls she paints and papers in bright floral prints she finds reassuring, giving her ownership, authority, a universe where she is in charge.

I have no such clarity. I move from one windowsill to another to get a different view. I stretch my yoga pad on the Berber carpet and lie on my back to catch trees at a new angle, a slice of shingled roof I don't usually see. I'm restless, caught in a kind of family quarrel between my body's need for a calm, gestational enclosure and the self's need for stimulation, engagement, expansion. Caught at that skirmish point writer and neurologist Oliver Sacks calls the "juncture of biology and biography." I have two dreams, one of a shelter crowded with people, all saved within its protective walls, the other of an enclosed room where everyone suffocates.

My immersion in the details of a room, in dust motes and dishes, carries an uneasy familiarity, not only of my mother's world, but of my own early marriage when, young and thoughtless, I agreed to leave a coveted Bay Area teaching job to accommodate my husband's career move to L.A., and was confined at home with a one-year-old. Truly confined. We lived in Beverly Glen Canyon, a narrow corridor with no bus service, and he took the car to work each day.

Except for a few glorious, windy days in the winter, when the sky was swept clean and everyone in the L.A. basin looked up in amazement to realize we were ringed by mountains to the east, smog hung in the air like ground mist. In the canyon, I could see the claustrophobic blanket lying above me, brown, particulate, unbreathable. One weekend, desperate for a fresh breath of air, I made my husband drive the three of us to those distant hazy mountains. We drove and drove, labored up the San Gabriel foothills and never left the smog behind.

I had believed marriage would launch me into a capacious adult world. Instead this world clamped me in. I wasn't one of those who disparaged domesticity. In fact, I enjoyed the stretch of quiet days with their small and ordinary contentments, baking fresh blueberry muffins, my daughter's bright eyes following me from her high chair. What rankled was the assumption that the home was my responsibility first and foremost, and I could have a career if it were convenient, if I could fit it in.

Mornings, after my husband sped away, I tidied and tended home, searing stew meat, hauling armloads of diapers to the damp basement laundry room strewn with lint and pennies, a humid, yeasty place beneath our house. In the hot afternoons, in the germinal, snatched hours when Lisa napped, I settled on the couch to read, speeding off on my own travels—to a place that would leave my husband and marriage behind. That was when the words of Germaine Greer and Betty Friedan caught my vague dissatisfactions and resentments in their sharp and brilliant light: I had become the invisible woman, marginalized, muted, public voice gone. Like so many women, my mind leapt to attention at this language for the unarticulated chafing I carried inside. I had planned to be in the restless, invigorating air of a classroom, not at home on the couch. More than anything, perhaps, I felt how easily I'd let myself fall into this domestic comfort hedged by limits.

Now here I am again. Somehow all the ameliorating years can't hold back the flood of inner doubts. I know in this postfeminist era we're supposed to be beyond those old tensions about staying home, beyond the idea of home as feminine space. Bill works at home, his computer and fax whirring and dinging in the next room. He vacuums and cooks. Still, those fears haunt me. The parallels are too strong, the old associations too difficult to dislodge. Women throughout history have been sent to a house and kept there: Rapunzel in her tower, women in a harem, nuns in a convent, a homemaker in the suburbs, or all the daughters of Eve who, as science writer Natalie Angier points out, "are not shut out of the garden but locked within it."[2]

Morbid thoughts. I remind myself of all the inventive women who, once ensconced, turned enclosure to their own purposes. Stories of religious women in the Middle Ages, Carmelite sisters who find in their seclusion and renunciation a vital autonomy and a strategy for an inner evolution toward "selfhood." For these women, feminist writer Carol Lee Flinders says, "enclosure, silence and the like no longer feel like preambles to extinction but preconditions for reclaiming their own wholeness."[3]

Or how about nineteenth-century English poet Christina Rossetti, who rejected marriage and declared herself unfit to be a governess, neatly curtailing anyone's claim on her. She spent most of her life in her family's London home, where, despite her strict Anglican piety, she wrote her thunderous verse, with its clamoring angels and mingling of erotic and religious fervor. Staying home allowed her to hold off the prescriptions of the outside world: get married, have children, don't be powerful, don't speak a woman's truth. Suffering was her theme, claim some critics. Personal independence, claim others. Christina, having burned her letters, leaves us to sort her meanings.

I remember an English professor of mine—we met in an old science lab and she always boosted herself up on the metal counter and lectured among beakers and sinks—beginning a talk about Rossetti by giving a shrug and dismissive laugh. "About her life, well, there's not much to say." I wagged my hand in the air and rattled on about the depth, activity, and range of the inner life, our cultural bias in favor of action over reflection, the way we overlook and render invisible the often raucous adventures of the spirit when the body appears tranquil or still. In fact, we have a long cultural history of retreat, from Moses to St. Aquinas to songwriter Leonard Cohen or writer Kathleen Norris: the spiritual seeker in crisis, the artist seeking inspiration and release from daily static, the harried mother in need of rejuvenation who pulls back from the demands of the profane to enter a transcendent, expansive space.

Despite my ardent defense of the internal life that day in my college English class, lying in bed groggy with fever, I have difficulty seeing myself in this tradition of retreat and renewal. I've stepped into a world out-of-sync with where I should be. Here I am still young but enacting the conversations of old age: zucchini softer please, and could you tuck the blanket over my feet? I had expected many more years of teaching and writing, of challenging conversations.

I'm cloistered in my uniform of illness, worn T-shirt and sweats, just as nuns don their habit and Rossetti her frumpy, unfashionable black dresses. I've fallen back into a life of enclosure, stung by the way the enforced confinement of illness mimics the restrictions and lack of choice women faced in earlier times. No wonder illness conjures the same polarized vision: home as salvation or prison.

There's another story of nineteenth-century female confinement, one jarringly familiar to a person with CFIDS. It goes like this: "I had her placed in a large, cheerful, airy room, with southern and eastern exposure, and directed that she should sleep alone. That every evening before retiring she should have a thorough rubbing and kneading of the muscles . . . and that just before the room was quiet for the night, she should have a glass of milk or a cup of beef tea, with a cracker as she tired of one or the other. Upon wakening she was to have a cup of Broma or Cocoa, and then to rest for half an hour. Then to have a sponge bath and brisk rubbing, after which rest in bed for nearly an hour. Then breakfast of some one of the many prepared grains as wheat germ, soft-boiled eggs, mutton chops or broiled beef steak, toast and butter, and a cup of coffee half cream. After breakfast rest in the sunshine. In the middle of the morning a glass of cold or hot milk, or a cup of beef-tea. Rest again."[4]

So read the physician instructions for a young woman of eighteen diagnosed as suffering from neurasthenia in 1885. She was prohibited from "all reading, writing and sewing and 'fancy work' but was permitted to do some light housework."[5] At an Iowa State Medical Association conference in 1886 the physician reported the patient responded well to this "rest cure" and "promises to have her health fully re-established."[6]

Isolation, bed rest, bland diet, careful supervision. It's impossible to miss the infantalizing trope or the eerie resonance with my own regime. At its extreme, the rest cure for the neurasthenic comprised an inhibiting routine in which the patient was not allowed to feed him- or herself or turn over in bed, but "must be fed by the nurse, and when he desires to change his position, he should be gently moved by the attendant. . . .

All source of mental and emotional excitement should be avoided. With this object in view, it is necessary to cut off, or strongly to advise the patient to cut off, communication with the outside world either absolutely or in a very large degree. This necessitates the exclusion of relatives and others, as well as the interruption of all correspondence. The patient, in other words, should be isolated, and the isolation should be rigid in proportion to the severity of the case."[7]

A large record of such stories exists. In the late nineteenth century, neurasthenia—characterized as an exhaustion of the nerves—was called "the disease of the age," with tens of thousands diagnosed, mostly women, in the United States and Western Europe. The thought of these stories fills me with unease. Was this a prescription for health or for controlling a group of mostly upper-middle-class women confronted with growing prospects, in an increasingly industrialized and modern world, of work and education?

Charlotte Perkins Gilman, nineteenth-century social critic and theorist, thought it was the latter. Fatigued and despondent after the birth of her daughter on March 23, 1885, Gilman consulted Silas Weir Mitchell, a Philadelphia nerve specialist. Mitchell was the infamous creator of the rest cure for neurasthenics; having discovered its benefits for Civil War soldiers fatigued from long marches, he applied it with vigor to all the men and women in his practice who he believed were exhausted from the incessant march of modern life. (Mitchell allowed modified versions of the cure for men, who he acknowledged would be less likely to accept such severe constraints.)

Here is Charlotte Perkins Gilman's acerbic account: "At that time the greatest nerve specialist in the country was Dr. S. W. Mitchell of Philadelphia. Through the kindness of a friend of Mr. Stetson's living in that city, I went to him and took 'the rest cure'; went with the utmost confidence, prefacing the visit with a long letter giving the 'history of the case' in a way a modern psychologist would have appreciated. Dr.

Mitchell only thought it proved self-conceit. He had a prejudice against the Beechers [prominent preachers and social reformers from whom Charlotte was descended]. 'I've had two women of your blood here already,' he told me scornfully. This eminent physician was well versed in two kinds of nervous prostration; that of the business man exhausted from too much work, and the society woman exhausted from too much play. The kind I had was evidently beyond him."[8]

A proper Victorian moralist, Mitchell subscribed to the idea that women's illnesses were linked to the stresses of higher education or social work, and that part of a physician's duty was to reeducate women as to their proper role, particularly as to the health benefits of running a household and rearing children. He was equally concerned that men remain firmly masculine. A novelist, Mitchell decried the proliferation of women writers in the literary magazines, claiming that the monthlies were becoming so feminized they would soon be menstruating.

Mitchell diagnosed Gilman with neurasthenia and prescribed a month of rich diet, absolute rest, and massage. He sent her home, admonishing her to "Live as domestic a life as possible. Have your child with you all the time. . . . Lie down an hour after each meal. Have but two hours' intellectual life a day. And never touch pen, brush or pencil as long as you live."[9]

Immortalized in Gilman's famous short story "The Yellow Wallpaper," about a woman who goes mad when her physician orders her confined for the sake of her health, Mitchell is the classic portrait of male authority demanding female submission. Writes Gilman, "I went home, followed those directions rigidly for months, and came perilously near to losing my mind."[10] Spiraling into deeper and deeper "mental agony," she realized the cure was the trap, her trust misplaced, the physician the problem. She got out of bed, divorced her husband, took up her pen, and returned to a life of lecturing, writing, and political activism for the rights of women, though for the rest of her life she suffered from a mental exhaustion ("my mind like a piece of boiled spinach") that cur-tailed her productivity.

In this story the woman who defies medical authority and the con-strictions and self-abnegating routine of the rest cure becomes a dynam-ic force for change, improving women's lives. She is the agent of her own recovery, incomplete though it is, a return rooted in defiance and refusal. Though she battles fatigue for the rest of her life, she rejects seclusion and she rejects submission, to the body or to medical authority.

I think about Gilman and her determined rebellion as I stare out the window at a pallid sky, a sling of vaporous clouds. This is the galling aspect of CFIDS: you defy it at your peril. I am confined, in bed, pre-cisely because of many years of defiance, day after month after year of refusing to let this illness define me, of putting on my city clothes and heading out the door, opening the opportunity, by whatever invidious mechanism, for the dysregulation in my immune or neuroendocrine system to be set in motion and do whatever it does that slams me back in bed. When I resist and disregard illness, I end up in its hold. Survival comes in acquiescence, or at least acceptance.

Despite this knowledge, a felt, bodily knowing from years of grind-ing experience, I still have fantasies of recovery that involve simply ris-ing from bed and striding out the door, refusing to submit, as if force of will could bring about some cellular magic. In this fantasy, my body has the capacity to revive, to overcome its deficit, and I see myself pacing along a hillside dirt trail as I used to. A breeze is on my face, and I'm moving through the world, strong-legged, in exhilarating forward motion.

I miss those winding trails, their dusty vegetative smell. One warm summer evening some years ago, probably in 1993, I had the urge to head up to the Strawberry Canyon trailhead for a sunset hike. I was tired and a bit achy, but I couldn't stand not being able to enjoy such a gor-geous evening, when the heat of the day hangs in warm pockets against the hills and the low sun casts a burnt-orange light across the Bay. Bill and I drove to the trailhead and started out, through an ivy-dense gorge, up a hairpin curve, past a stretch of fragrant eucalyptus, to a brilliant Bay view. The next day I was extra fatigued and foggy, my brain turned to slush. The day after, I had that all over fluish feeling and could barely walk a few blocks. It took me six weeks to recover. Postexertional malaise is the technical term—when exercise or doing too much provokes a flare-up of symptoms or excessive fatigue. I call it paying for my fun. I no longer have even that option.

No one knows for sure what causes this postexertional malaise. One theory is that a mitochondrial dysfunction in the cells means the body doesn't produce energy the way it should. Another theory links the problem to an immune system defect in an enzyme called RNase-L that in turn produces poor oxidative metabolism, which means people get fatigued more easily during exercise. Others have suggested that malfunctions in the autonomic nervous system result in decreased blood flow to the brain and muscle tissues, compromising the ability to exercise. Some investigators have postulated that cardiac insufficiency is at the root of CFIDS. Unexplored heart problems may cause the heart to pump abnormally, resulting in postexertional symptoms that parallel those of heart failure patients. One exercise physiologist claims that when a CFIDS patient takes an exercise test, the results look like those of a patient with cardiovascular or pulmonary disease.[11]

There's been tremendous debate within CFIDS circles about whether to treat CFIDS with graded exercise—gradually trying to increase one's exercise program—or whether postexertional malaise makes this impossible or counterproductive. Many persons with CFIDS (PWCs) are adamant that those who champion graded exercise don't understand the biological nature of CFIDS and are advancing the misguided notion that CFIDS can be cured through force of will: If you would just get up on that exercise treadmill, you could work your way to better health. This line of thinking implies the enervation of CFIDS is similar to that of someone who is deconditioned, an assumption that ignores the science on severe physiological dysfunction in CFIDS patients.

Dr. Anthony Komaroff sets the debate in perspective: "I think the literature demonstrates some patients respond well [to exercise] and others clearly do not respond well, suggesting that there are subsets of patients among those with CFS. A universal rule is unlikely to apply to all patients."[12] Dr. Komaroff's comment reflects the growing recognition of the need to subtype patients in order to better understand the biological processes at work. His words also reinforce the inadequacy of the current Fukuda case definition for CFS, which casts an overly wide net. In Great Britain and Canada, postexertional fatigue is one of the major criteria for myalgic encephalomyelitis (ME), whereas the 1994 Fukuda definition for CFS lists it as one of the eight minor criteria.[13] Since a patient needs to exhibit only four of the eight minor criteria to be diagnosed with CFS, postexertional fatigue is much less central to the U.S. case definition, and this results in a more varied group of patients who meet the definition. Many CFIDS advocates argue that postexertional fatigue is a hallmark of this disease and should be one of the major criteria for diagnosis.

Until we better understand the mechanism of this illness, most people familiar with CFIDS continue to advocate the "envelope theory" of exercise as the best road to improved health: stay within your energy envelope by keeping your available energy and expended energy in line. Do as much as you feel able, but not more, so your body can slowly heal. Says general practitioner Dr. Marsha Wallace, "The key is to avoid doing anything for which there is significant 'payback,' even over the next several days."[14]

So here I am. My energy envelope, this February of 1996, translates to twenty-three quiet hours a day in my bedroom, and an hour or so of light activity around the house. It's maddening to think I've become the enforcer of Dr. Mitchell's stultifying regime—Dr. Diet and Dr. Quiet, he was called—with my regulated routine of healthy meals and rest. Oatmeal, banana, and soy milk at seven A.M. Shower and rest. Chicken noodle soup with greens at nine. Hot compresses and steam. Relaxation tapes for an hour. More rest. Broiled chicken, steamed potatoes, zucchini, and applesauce at eleven.

I exert tremendous control over my body, or rather, it controls me, and like it or not, I have to obey this internalized authority. I have to struggle to see in self-control and denial the tools of health, which of course they are, and to disentangle the tentacles of repression from the assertion of self-care. Health lies in relinquishing activity, altering ambition, foregoing the streets. I have to leave fiery protest to others, to those, like Gilman, who can gather the strength. I have to imagine I'm protesting in a different way, protesting the ethic of continual striving, blind ambition, and ignoring the body's needs.

Charlotte Perkins Gilman sounds a lament familiar to anyone with CFIDS, recounting what happened when she pushed herself beyond her limits. "The result has been a lasting loss of power, total in some directions, partial in others; the necessity for a laboriously acquired laziness foreign to both temperament and conviction, a crippled life.

"But since my public activities do not show weakness, nor my writings, and since brain and nerve disorder is not visible, short of lunacy or literal 'prostration,' this lifetime of limitation and wretchedness, when I mention it, is flatly disbelieved. When I am forced to refuse invitations, to back out of work that seems easy, to own that I cannot read a heavy book, apologetically alleging this weakness of mind, friends gibber amiably, 'I wish I had your mind!' I wish they had, for a while, as a punishment for doubting my word. What confuses them is the visible work I have been able to accomplish. They see activity, achievement, they do not see blank months of idleness; nor can they see what the work would have been if the powerful mind I had to begin with had not broken at twenty-four."[15]

By 1910, twenty-five years after Gilman was subjected to S. Weir Mitchell's moralizing, neither her postpartum depression nor her persistent fatigue would have been diagnosed as neurasthenia. The term was falling out of favor. As one reviewer of a book on neurasthenia proclaimed, "Neurasthenic disorders are a bit out of fashion at the present day."[16]

Neurasthenia Revised

I knew neither peace nor comfort night nor day. There remained all
the usual pain of nerve trunks of peripheral nerve endings, the exquisite sensitiveness of body, the inability to bear a touch heavier than the
brush of a butterfly's wing, the insomnia, lack of strength . . . the
inability to use my brain at my study and writing as I wished.
—Margaret Cleaves, *The Autobiography Of A Neurasthene: As Told By
One Of Them And Recorded By Margaret A. Cleaves, M.D.*

In her 1910 autobiography, Margaret Cleaves, a self-proclaimed
"essential neurasthene" (which she distinguished from those
"symptomatic" neurasthenes whose complaints were a matter of overindulgence and coddling, and whose neurotic grievances sullied the reputation of genuine sufferers such as Cleaves), records a fascinating story
of neurasthenia, an illness characterized by "lack of nerve force" that was
widely diagnosed in America and Western Europe between 1880 and
1910. Reading Cleaves's account, the story of a hardworking, dedicated,
chronically ill physician in New York City, I can't help but get an uncanny sense of déjà vu, and I'm not alone. A number of researchers have
suggested that CFS is "neurasthenia revived," as the symptoms, illness
course, and unclear biological basis present an eerie correspondence.[1]

To someone like myself, Cleaves's words are striking in their familiarity. "The suffering of the essential neurasthene is not imaginary by
any means. It is as real as the pain from a fractured bone. But because of
the absence of anatomic lesions or a pathological anatomy, the patho-

logical physiology is ignored in an estimate of the physical suffering and mental torment endured and its genuineness questioned."[2] To read Cleaves's tale is to wonder. Is her "inability to bear a touch heavier than the brush of a butterfly's wing" (Yes!) the same as mine? Is there some familial connection between her debilities and my own?

Her descriptions display a remarkable resemblance: "I had so little physical strength that to hold a newspaper was a weariness, let alone a book."[3] Or this: "The sense of cerebral and spinal exhaustion was extreme, and to make it all worse there was congestion of the sensory cortex which made me intolerant of the vibrations of light and sound, in fact—the external world—but I could not get away from them."[4]

Her book brims with exhortations to the self to remain strong, complaints about how little others understand, and determination to find through discipline and meaningful work a satisfying life. Over and over the similarities are there: The frustration of an uncomprehending physician: "My physician believed most thoroughly in exercise and I was directed to take bicycle lessons, and as soon as possible got out into the open. Here is where mistakes are apt to be made in the care of neurasthenic patients. . . . I obeyed although I fell off my wheel from sheer exhaustion again and again. The result was disastrous. I should have been counselled to spend every hour not needed for my duties in a hammock, preferably out of doors."[5] The hard-won lessons: "The only opportunity for better conditions than these is to be found in a strict observance of the neurasthene's golden rule, never to go beyond the point of fatigue."[6] The invisibility of her condition to others and the frustration of a limited life: "The observer only reads that which spells success and knows naught of the long weary hours of pain and disability without achievement of any sort."[7]

After years of pushing herself, Cleaves collapsed, then with huge doses of self-care improved, only to spiral down again. Finally, an ill-advised trip to France pushed her over the edge, a trip her doctor assured her she could manage. She lived the rest of her days in a state of fluctuating exhaustion and pain, devoted nonetheless to her patients and work.

I'm treading controversial waters to entertain the idea that CFIDS finds a mirror in neurasthenia. CFIDS sufferers hotly contest the association between CFS and neurasthenia, since, after its two- or three-decade heyday, neurasthenia came to be widely discredited and equated with emotional disorders. By the early 1900s, medical textbooks and periodicals were rife with statements such as "neurotic, neurasthenic, hysterical and hypochondriacal are, on the lips of the majority of clinical teachers, terms of opprobrium," or "all neurasthenic states are in reality depression—perhaps minor, attenuated, atypical masked, but always forms of anxious melancholia."[8] If illnesses are judged by the company they keep, neurasthenia is not good company. The authors of one article exploring the CFS-neurasthenia link argue, "Chronic fatigue syndrome will meet the same fate as neurasthenia—a decline in social value as it is demonstrated that the majority of its sufferers are experiencing primary psychiatric disorders or psychophysiological reactions and that the disorder is often a culturally sanctioned form of illness behavior."[9] In this context, to claim CFIDS as an incarnation of neurasthenia is to demean and dismiss.

I think, though, that our view of neurasthenia is ripe for revision. When the flap over ascribing to CFIDS a disreputable lineage is set aside, putting these distant cousins in the same room can open an intriguing conversation—not about the foibles and inadequacies of patients, but about the deficiencies and limits of the medical system these patients confront. The controversy surrounding both neurasthenia and CFIDS points to deep-seated inadequacies in our Western concept of illness and disease—in particular, the artificial mind/body division, the impact of specialization, and the narrow categories available to describe complex, chronic, multicausal illnesses.

To delve into past epidemics is to dive into speculation and conjecture. Really, it's a moot point to ask if CFS is the modern neurasthenia, since it's difficult to compare earlier clinical accounts with modern data: case definitions are different and not uniformly applied, records are haphazard and often subjective, populations live(d) under different conditions, and pathogens themselves are mutable, unstable entities. Medical historians compile their records from doctors' accounts, patient diaries, newspaper articles, public documents, medical texts. What does all this data tell us? It's unclear. Records are skewed by class (those who couldn't afford doctors aren't included), by literacy (the illiterate didn't keep diaries), by physician bias (S. Weir Mitchell in 1881 described his chronically fatigued female patients as "the pests of many households, who constitute the despair of physicians"[10]), and by the medical limits and perspectives of the time (minor depression, for instance, was not readily recognized in the late 1800s). If we read the accounts of a doctor making his living from "sofa cases," as wealthy invalid women were called in the late nineteenth century, what can we deduce from his records? How much should we generalize from them? On the basis of a doctor's report of clinical symptoms, can we determine a specific diagnosis?

It seems reasonable to assume there have always been fatiguing illnesses and postinfectious syndromes. Researcher and internist Dr. Dedra Buchwald points to a two-thousand-year-old Chinese medical text that refers to symptoms very similar to CFIDS.[11] In the 1730s the Scottish physician George Cheyne used the term "English Malady" to describe the nervous disorder he felt was at the heart of many chronic illnesses. Cheyne believed the English Malady to be a condition of the cultivated upper classes, and attributed it to leisure, refined sensibilities, and excess. His conclusions are no surprise: Cheyne himself suffered from the illness, at one time weighing in at four hundred fifty pounds from gourmet overindulgence.[12]

But it was in the late nineteenth century that records of fatigue mushroomed, and neurasthenia, which had been mentioned earlier in scattered cases, became "the disease of the age." The American neurologist George Miller Beard solidified the term "neurasthenia" as a clinical entity in his 1869 article, "Neurasthenia, or Nervous Exhaustion."[13] Beard defined neurasthenia as "an impoverishment of nervous force,"[14] a description that for all its scientific trappings rings with vitalistic echoes, as in weak *chi* or not enough *prana*.

Beard gathered under the term neurasthenia a protean and wide-flung list of complaints, which he acknowledged—with a poet's appreciation for ambiguity—were "slippery, fleeting and vague."[15] Yet as a man with a grand vision, he insisted they were one disease. His 1881 book *American Nervousness* listed two pages of symptoms—a list, he assured readers, that was not exhaustive—including: insomnia, flushing, drowsiness, bad dreams, cerebral irritation, dilated pupils, pain, pressure and heaviness in the head, noises in the ears, mental irritability, tenderness of the teeth and gums, nervous dyspepsia, pains in the back, heaviness of the loins and limbs, shooting pains, cold hands and feet, pain in the feet, special idiosyncrasies in regard to food, medicines, and external irritants, local spasms of muscles, convulsive movements, especially on going to sleep, cramps, a feeling of profound exhaustion and on and on.[16]

Beard knew what he was describing. He himself suffered as a young man from classic neurasthenic symptoms: nervousness, lack of vitality, indigestion, ringing in the ears, pains in the side, and morbid fears.[17] Born in Montville, Connecticut, in 1839 to a pious Congregational couple, Beard had been pressured to follow his father's path into the ministry and was torn by inner conflict. The man who would later become his medical partner, A. D. Rockwell, paints a picture of the young Beard as "worried about his soul," someone who on his gloomy Sunday walks along Manhasset Bay, Long Island, "deplores the wickedness" of the young people sailing and fishing on the Lord's day.[18] A photo of Beard shows a serious man with narrow lips, high forehead, brooding eyes, a thin cover of straight hair, and mutton-chop sideburns, looking nothing like the self-promoting zealot he would become.

Ultimately Beard rejected the pulpit, subsequently recovering from his years of poor health, to preach the moral lessons of the body. Repudiating the dogmatic strictures of his upbringing, he graduated from Columbia's College of Physicians and Surgeons in 1866 and became an evangelist of an objective medical science. He developed a rabid antipathy to the wave of spiritualism and mysticism engaging the popular imagination and championed the materialist views that informed late-nineteenth-century medicine, views that proclaimed diease to have an observable, physical basis.[19]

In some ways a bland character—singularly focused on science, temperamentally mild despite an apparent egotism—Beard becomes colorful if only because of the force of his beliefs and his fearlessness in presenting them, over and over and over. Beard had, writes Rockwell, "a settled conviction that the surest way to establish the truth, as he understood it, was boldly and persistently to reiterate it."[20] As if to convince himself as well.

From today's perspective, Beard and other neurologists of his time, these adamantly scientific men, seem able to hold remarkably fluid concepts of illness. Since the Civil War and the recognition of nervous exhaustion in soldiers, neurology, which previously had focused on physical disorders of the brain and nervous system such as epilepsy or paralysis, had evolved to include emotional or mental symptoms, such as insomnia, depression, or nervousness. By the early twentieth century these symptoms would be seen as psychogenic—originating in the mind though expressed in the body—and wrested away by the developing field of psychiatry. But Beard practiced in a transitional time, before the rise of psychiatry and high-tech medicine, in which these ambiguous late-Victorian nervous conditions were treated under the aegis of a somatic, scientific medicine.

Like other Victorian neurologists, Beard believed that the vague, often outlandish complaints of his patients—complaints he knew only too well—had a somatic basis, despite the absence of a readily discernible organic lesion. Neurasthenia, Beard held, was just as much a material phenomenon as typhoid or cholera, but one science couldn't yet fully describe. "I feel assured that [neurasthenia] will in time be substantially confirmed by microscopical and chemical examinations of those patients who died in a neurasthenic condition."[21]

With Darwinian fervor, he believed neurasthenia was the necessary price we paid for our advances as a civilization, and a distinctly "American malady." The same finely tuned nervous system that produced higher civilization was unfortunately susceptible to its stress. A reflection of the class, sex, and race bias of the time, neurasthenia was cast as a disease of the refined, professional classes, affecting as many men as women; in fact, 10 percent of Beard's patients were other doctors. In men, however, neurasthenia was said to be caused by mental fatigue and overwork; in women, it was attributed to reproductive stresses. The difficulty raised by the fact that working-class people were also diagnosed with the disorder was dispensed with by attributing their weakness to debauchery and drink. Beard scoffed at the idea that a "Congo Negro" could suffer from neurasthenia.

By invoking the language of nerves rather than the language of the psyche, Beard spared sufferers of these conditions—who otherwise would have been diagnosed as having hypochondria, hysteria, or melancholia—the stigma and indignity of mental illness. A somatic diagnosis meant acceptance and sympathy from doctors, family, and friends, and the possibility of treatment. Beard believed he could cure patients through diet, rest, and electrotherapy, and enthusiastically applied galvanized electric currents to patients' eye sockets, temples, necks, and spines. When he once cured a man with this treatment even though the galvanic battery was dead, Beard added "definite expectation" (later to be called "suggestion") to his list of curative therapies.

Beard rooted neurasthenia in the physical, but he gave it a social etiology, attributing the rise in nervous ailments to the fast pace of modern life. In particular he cited "steam power, the periodical press, the telegraph, the sciences, and the mental activity of women."[22] In an American age of accomplishment, of thermodynamics, steam power, and electricity, the circuits, Beard pronounced, were overloaded. He compared lack of nerve force to an overdrawn bank account or dimming lamps, finding in the advancing fields of economics and physics the metaphors of exhaustion. "The force in this nervous system . . . is limited; and when new functions are interposed in the circuit, as modern civilization is constantly requiring us to do, there comes a period, sooner or later, varying in different individuals, and at different times of life, when the amount of force is insufficient to keep all the lamps actively burning; those that are weakest go out entirely, or, as more frequently happens, burn faint and feebly—they do not expire, but give an insufficient and unstable light."[23]

A man of science who went on faith, who incorporated vitalistic principles into the metaphors of modern science, who both appreciated and tried to corral ambiguity, Beard seems to exemplify the tensions and contradictions between the somatic theory of late-nineteenth-century medicine and the wayward, insubordinate bodies of actual patients. The diagnosis of neurasthenia filled a nebulous space in which scientific certitude proved elusive, the body unreliable, and the physician's practice ambiguous. Neurasthenia retained a mercurial essence; cultural critic Walter Benjamin would later cast the neurasthenic body as a corporeal text, "a living image open to all kinds of revision by the interpretive artist," usually a physician, whose diagnosis "stabilized the chaos of appearances."[24] Despite his paternalistic projection of the physician as grand decoder of the body, Benjamin captures the confusion and anarchy at the heart of neurasthenia.

Beard's somatic diagnosis conferred on patients legitimacy and respectability, and gave physicians a diagnosis and treatments for perplexing symptoms. But by the early twentieth century this malleable diagnostic space was being dismantled. As science revealed the biological basis of an increasing number of conditions, such as lead poisoning or Addison's disease, and as Freudian theories of neurosis took hold, Beard's diagnostic category could not cohere. Neurasthenic complaints were seen as a "mob of incoherent symptoms borrowed from the most diverse disorders"[25] and attributed to either an underlying, previously unrecognized disease or to psychoneurosis. Beard's fervent belief that the scientific basis of neurasthenia would eventually be revealed was turned on its head; scientific advance delineated other illnesses and in so doing eviscerated neurasthenia.

Today neurasthenia is seen to occupy a temporary historical space during which science demanded a physical basis for illness but hadn't yet discerned the organic underpinnings of many diseases, and before the idea of psychogenic ailments was solidified. Beard is recognized mainly as a neurologist who, in advance of Freud, acknowledged environmental and social factors in stress and mental illness. In other words, any disease that is truly organic has been peeled away from the term "neurasthenia," and what's left are the psychoneuroses. For all Beard's efforts, in the United States the term has been not only rejected but restigmatized.[26]

Beard would turn over in his grave. Until his premature death of pneumonia in 1883, he was a relentless promoter of his ideas and reputation. Proselytizing and grandstanding—he's been accused of being the

Barnum of American medicine—rehashing his "discoveries" in an end-less series of papers, he strove to convince the public and the medical establishment of the validity of his construct.

Beard's reputation for bombast seems well earned. In the Preface to his 1881 *American Nervousness: Its Causes and Consequences* he justifies his endless republication of the same material as refinement and development of his ideas.[27] He decries the lack of professional attention and acceptance for his discoveries, and particularly that his "graduating thesis," which first laid out his work, "not only received no prize, but not even an honorable mention."[28] He laments that the public won't accept his ideas. He attacks as "delusion" his detractors' idea that nervous disorders, if observed properly, would have been found in previous times and other cultures, an argument that undermined Beard's central contention that neurasthenia was new, American first and foremost, and a product of advanced society. He dismisses his critics as Johnny-come-latelies who are so wedded to the status quo they can't see original, cutting-edge work for what it is: "[I]n all our cyclopedias of medicine . . . one shall look vainly—save here and there, for an intelligent and differential description of neurasthenia, the most frequent, the most important, the most interesting disease of our time, or of any time."[29] He can't resist that last self-aggrandizing pronouncement, "or of any time."

Ah, poor neglected neurasthenia and its unfairly unrecognized champion. Poor Beard, whose untimely death prevented him from living to see neurasthenia become widely accepted and discussed, as it was from roughly 1880 to 1910. He would seem an unlikely person to resurrect, not the kind you'd want as an associate. And yet. . . .

Beard's story fascinates me because of the parallels between that turn-of-the-century period and our own as we grapple with the vagaries of the body and the limits of science. As with Beard's neurasthenics, those of us with CFIDS exist in an obscure, interim, transitional space.

Like Beard, we place our faith in modern science and wait for it to dissect and explain our illness. But perhaps looking to the wisdom and power of biomedical knowledge alone to solve the riddle of CFIDS is short-sighted, just as dismissing Beard's neurasthenia as the misguided conjuring of prescientific knowledge is too facile. Was Beard, with his belief in progress and science, grappling with something he couldn't recognize? Will there always be something about the complex processes of mind and body that are irreducible to the binary schema of modern science?

What intrigues me about Beard's neurasthenia is the model it offers for understanding illness as a complex interplay of mind, body, and environment, what many today would call a biopsychosocial or biocultural model. Trailing the rank odor of racism, sexism, and nationalistic hype, Beard's neurasthenia nonetheless offered a multicausal explanation for illness and a holistic view in which psyche and soma were linked. Not yet confined by the reductionism of twentieth-century biological science or the post-Freudian split between mind and body, Beard and other practitioners of his day could accommodate the plasticity and complexity of their patients' disorders. They legitimized clinical symptoms without laboratory confirmation and thus recouped those with poorly understood complaints into the medical system, where they were treated rather than spurned.

And here's a key: When the neurasthenic bubble burst, it took with it, ragtag as it might have been, a descriptive umbrella that accommodated the perspectives of both patients and professionals. Patients and physicians alike viewed the patient's symptoms as organically based. By the early twentieth century, when this accord disintegrated, it was the patient's reliability that was questioned. One writer on neurasthenia, cultural historian Tom Lutz, homes in on this crucial shift. He quotes F. G. Gosling, who reiterates the oft-noted fact that as doctors became more knowledgeable about neurasthenia they "perceived important dissimilarities among so-called neurasthenics."[30] Lutz goes on to say: "What this doesn't explain, of course, is why, after almost a half century, these differences and difficulties became perceived not as puzzles to be solved but as proof that the paradigm should be abandoned."[31] Bingo.

The same observation could be made of CFIDS critics who dismiss CFIDS as a wastebasket diagnosis, insisting the assortment and profusion of symptoms prove its unreliability. Why is patient heterogeneity, the variety of symptoms across the patient population, used to discredit an illness rather than being seen as "a puzzle to be solved," perhaps suggesting the need to subgroup patients or to revise the case definition? Why is it the patients who are questioned rather than the existing paradigm of disease?

Those of us who display symptoms for which the physical cause is not firmly delineated have always been a fly in the ointment of a materialist science. Physicians don't know what to do with us, and we don't know where to go ourselves. To claim for CFIDS a social or emotional component risks stigmatization and diverts attention from the need for medical research. Yet to force our illness into the biomedical mold may eclipse its complexity and draw focus away from social and environmental causes. Researchers have observed that CFIDS patients often offer a more holistic, multifactorial explanation of their illness than do the medical practitioners they see.[32]

Lutz sees in the diagnosis of neurasthenia a linguistic and medical bridge between soma and psyche, a middle way to understand illness that avoids the either/or construct of physical or psychological disease. Acknowledging this interim, murky space, rather than being misguided, can be seen as a gesture toward defying the artificial division between mental and physical illness, a creative way to reconfigure the rigid boundaries of medical specialties and fashion a more fluid, holistic space for illness. It's a gesture that is still much needed today.

Interestingly, physicians and researchers are now actively debating how to subtype CFS patients—perhaps by similar symptoms or illness history, or by the predominant organ system involved—to make both treatment and research more effective. And as of this writing, the CDC is working to revise the 1994 Fukuda case definition to make it a better tool for selecting those with CFS.

As the diagnosis of neurasthenia fell into disrepute, I suspect there remained a core group (the "essential neurasthenes," to use Margaret Cleaves's emphatic term) whose symptoms could not be attributed to previously unrecognized illnesses or the psychoneuroses. It's this undeciphered third category that interests me, a cluster that most likely included occult medical disorders and postinfectious syndromes. Those of us with CFIDS are the occulted bodies in today's high-tech landscape. We live in that ambiguous space biomedicine still can't explain. And we're still in need of a champion who can offer a multicausal, holistic model of illness within the accepted corridors of medicine.

For all Beard's hankering after medical legitimacy, his "American nervousness," that expression of cultural advance and nationalistic pride, may rumble with undercurrents of dissent and resistance against the medical establishment and the materialist thinking of his day. I can't help thinking of Beard's radical conversion from religious conflict to scientific clarity. Such swings in dogmatic conviction usually say more about submerged conflict than certitude. In his autobiography *Rambling Recollections,* Beard's medical partner A. D. Rockwell raised his own questions about the force of Beard's beliefs. "The pendulum which had swung so long in one direction made an equal arc in the other. While giving up every vestige of belief in the supernatural, he might have made more of the soul of man and of human emotion and sentiment. Nothing seemed to interest him much in literature or books but pure science, accuracy of statement, mathematical precision or certainty."[33] Rockwell's insight that a pendulum swinging too far in one direction ends up in a one-dimensional realm applies as well to the materialist biomedicine that shapes medical thinking today.

8

Remedies, Advice, and the (Dis)Information Glut

Dear Madame,
I try every remedy sent to me. I am now on number 87. Yours is number 2,653. I am looking forward to its beneficial results.

—Mark Twain, quoted in Albert Bigelow Paine, *Mark Twain: A Biography*, Vol. III, Part 2

February 1996

I'm fortunate that among my neighbors are a number of passionate gardeners. I don't have to go farther than the sidewalk to view lavish banks of powdery calla lilies with their swanlike necks, masses of decorative rose-pink and red camellias, and vigorous stands of rhododendron with their frilly white bouquets. Even the scruffy yards have an exuberant energy, overrun by the wild ferocity of plants that will have their way—climbing roses smothering a shed, invading jungles of saucer-sized nasturtium leaves.

I'm out this late February day for my short walk, inhaling this vitality like a drug. The weather has warmed and a ripple of new, momentary energy propels my ten-minute foray outside. I've managed to walk three houses up the block for several weeks now, two or three times a week.

I decide to make my way across the street for a change of scenery and to admire a brilliant swath of yellow daffodils in a neighbor's front yard. Behind a screen of twiggy wisteria bramble, I can see this neighbor pulling dead shoots from her winter bulbs. In that odd way of urban life, where a street can be an invisible barrier, she and I have barely exchanged a few words, though we've lived across from each other for almost fifteen years. A small woman, she wears a bulky workcoat over cocoa-brown pants. I weigh for a moment whether to take the bold step of saying hello, a strain on my throat. I measure out my whispery talking as if it were gold, which it is, saving it for my closest family. But on this sunny afternoon I can't resist the prospect of an ordinary encounter, a neighborly chat. The chance for idle chatter takes on the aura of a hugely wonderful treat.

She seems startled by my low-voiced greeting, pulling herself up with a grimace and limping along a narrow path of brick-orange flagstones to the sidewalk. I tell her how much I enjoy her dense plantings of bulbs, now knuckling their way through the hard winter earth. Lemony daffodils and paper whites. Buttercream freesias ladling their perfumed scent into the air.

"Do you do all this yourself?" I gesture broadly.

"Used to, but I hurt my foot laying flagstones in the driveway. Now I hire someone."

I commiserate. "I can't walk very far, either. I have chronic fa—"

"—fatigue syndrome." She finishes my sentence, regarding me skeptically. She seems to know I have CFS, as if the neighborhood were sprouting tangled, suspicion-filled rumors.

Before I can say a word, she plows ahead with the all-too-familiar drumbeat of someone out to save my soul. "A friend of mine had that. She was really helped by acupuncture. Have you seen that new book about chronic fatigue at Cody's?"

I shake my head.

"It's in the window. You should get it. There's lots of books about that." Her eyes narrow. "Do you know that acupuncturist on College Avenue?"

"On College?"

"It's really close. You could walk up there."

"I can't really walk that far."

"You could get someone to drive you."

"I did acupuncture last fall. It didn't really help." Bill had hauled me into a nearby office in those terrible fall months. It had been a disaster, the whole exertion making me worse, not better.

She sputters on, fully revved, "My friend was really helped by her . . . ," then eyes me sternly. "There's help out there if you want it." With that she turns on her heels and hobbles up her wisteria-strung front porch, shutting the green wooden door behind her.

I'm stunned. What I thought would be a recaptured moment of normalcy, a casual exchange over a flower bed, has left me chastised like a recalcitrant child. I don't have the strength to follow her up the steps, can't talk further. I'm not up to writing a note or trying to sort things out with a neighbor I hardly know. I have to leave that misunderstanding and rancor hanging in the air and go back to bed.

These are the moments when my isolation and impotence bring a sharp, stifled anger. The presumption of other people who don't know me, don't know my history with this illness, don't know much, if anything, about CFS, never ceases to amaze me. And to have this prized moment of sunshine and blossoms turned into another frustrating misconnection is doubly stinging.

Fortunately, not everyone is so quick to judgment as this proselytizing neighbor. Most people shift into that gear I call "lovingly anxious." There's something about the state of illness, especially an illness with no known cause or cure, that stirs the impulse to hand me or Bill little slips of paper with names of doctors, homeopaths, special lozenges, Chinese herbs, megavitamin formulas. The reflexive urge to offer a remedy or solution in the face of my feebleness is something I'm becoming used to. Even Bill, normally the king of skeptics, is not immune. Last week he burst through our front door and announced in the triumphant tone of someone with the winning lottery number, "Magnets!"

He'd been away for six days visiting his eighty-three-year-old mother in Florida, having put off the trip while he nursed me through the fall. Her health had been shaky for a while, but she was in better shape than he had feared. He seemed reinvigorated, and genuinely hopeful that he had hit on a solution to our quagmire.

"Magnets?"

He set his suitcases beside him in the middle of the living room, where I was draped on the couch, and launched into his story. The attendant on his flight swore by magnets for her aching feet and wore them in her shoes. He had stood in the rumbling hull thirty thousand feet above earth while she stuffed magnets in his running shoes and pressed on his buoyant, outstretched arms to demonstrate the magnets' force field.

With this, he pantomimed, taking a stiff-armed scarecrow stance next to the bamboo and glass coffee table. On the basis of the flight attendant's effusive claims to have cured her father's insomnia, he was poised to dash out and buy me a mattress cover with magnets weighing it down like rocks. "What can it hurt?"

When magnets evoked in me the enthusiasm of a refrigerator, Bill boomed, "Well, then, how about Udo's oil?"

There must be something about the instant intimacy of travel that induces people to trade personal health tonics like favorite recipes. The van driver who had just delivered Bill from the airport, weaving through rush hour traffic, had raved about the healing properties of this magic elixir. The driver claimed he'd been sick and tired all the time and now felt invigorated by a youthful energy. Other oils wouldn't do, he insisted. Only Udo's had the perfect formula.

The next day Bill arrived home from our local health food store and extracted from a brown bag with great flourish a thick blue bottle.

Wielding a spoon, he downed a hefty tablespoon of brown, gluey fluid. "Yuck!"

I declined to join him.

Undeterred, and not about to waste his money, Bill faithfully imbibed this serum until a few days later, poking through Muenster cheeses and calamari olives at the market, he spied the van driver standing guard by the refrigerated oils like a sidewalk evangelist, pitching his remedy to whoever would listen.

Talk of Udo's oil evaporated, but not of magnets. The magnet company must strategically court its salespeople among those whose line of work offers them a captive audience. The next time Bill found himself in a reclining leather chair with a mouthful of dental equipment, the hygienist poking his molars and incisors, face inches from his, rhapsodized nonstop about how her father's sleep problems had been miraculously cured by Japanese magnet therapy. She was a salesperson for the same company as the airline flight attendant.

As many ill people are, I have been astounded and touched, annoyed and angered, by the pervasive urge to provide a solution and the fervor of each person's belief in his or her chosen panacea, each different. This outpouring, offered with a can-do optimism, seems yet another trivialization, another signal of how little other people understand the magnitude and severity of this illness. It seems another measure of my aloneness, as if that extra battery charge that lets a healthy person maintain a 24/7 life is all I must need, too. Worse, I can't talk, let alone rouse the energy to respond. No, this is serious. This is Bigtime. It's beyond salts and mushrooms and herbs.

Over time, my irritation has mixed with resignation and amusement. I sometimes think of my illness as an imaginative spur, like those creativity exercises about how many different ways you can use a brick. How many ways can we think of to get Dorothy well? In the course of my illness I've been offered the following suggestions, probably a tame list compared to those of some with CFIDS: exercise, lie on the ground, blood transfusion, vitamin B$_{12}$ injections, electric current therapy, check for parasites, lift weights, see a therapist, consult a psychic healer, Udo's oil, Tahitian Noni, bovine colostrum, propolis, Prozac, goldenseal, move to the country, Ayurvedic medicine, medical qi gong, thyroid pills, Ennerprime, salt, no-carbohydrate diet, human growth hormone, ozone therapy, Japanese magnet therapy. Somewhere between the blood transfusion and the magnets I've become a little jaded. It's no wonder the eminent Boston neurosurgeon of the early twentieth century, Harvey Cushing, once noted, "The task of the physician is to protect the patient from the patient's relatives so that nature can heal him."

I've had to hold most friends and family at bay, too exhausted to deal with them. Lisa has been handling the calls, the worried inquiries. Five months and she's still in bed? I scribble her a message: tell them to write me a note or leave a phone message. I want to hear from them, but from a distance.

My brain can't handle more effort, more commotion, more swarming and tending, more personality, more questions, more words, more slant-eyed glances. More Ideas for How to Get Better. I can feel everyone encouraging me on, hoping I can find the right pill, the magic remedy. To me it feels like trying to grieve in a hurry, going through Kübler-Ross's stages of grief lickety-split so you can get back to your tennis game. I know that isn't going to happen. That's not the way grief works, nor CFIDS.

Perhaps you have to be on the other side of this remedy barrage to feel its full import. Home remedies, nostrums, and purgatives are as old as illness, but today's remedies and cures are a rampant, corporate-driven incarnation of the old sidewalk hawkers, promoted by a sophisticated multibillion-dollar pharmaceutical and alternative health industry.

These industries bombard us with commercial messages—especially since 1999, when Congress voted to allow direct advertising to consumers—that both prey upon and shape cultural attitudes about illness: if something's wrong, we can fix it.

It's a message with deep roots in the American concept of self-improvement. We want to believe we can heal ourselves through pills, treatments, or attitudinal shifts, and we pump billions of dollars a year into an industry eager to meet our needs. Those books on CFIDS? Along with lots of good information are long lists of suggested remedies, beginning with Acetyl-L-carnitine and Acyclovir, working their way through nasal douching and nitroglycerin, to Xanax and Zoloft—hundreds and hundreds of alternative and pharmaceutical interventions. If it's a cure for fatigue, and even if it's not, it's hyped for CFIDS. The acupuncturist I went to in the early 1990s, when my health was going steadily downhill, used to tell stories about patients coming into his office with shopping bags full of their pills and herbs. "The first thing I'd do," he said, "is tell them to empty that bag."

While promoters promise "natural" cures designed to strengthen our innate healing abilities, in reality the commodification of illness works against our basic faith in the body. Individually, some remedies can be useful. In the aggregate, such commercialization urges holistic remedies on us so massively and indiscriminately as to increase our alienation from our bodies and take us further from Hippocrates' timeless wisdom: the natural healing force within each one of us is the greatest force in getting well.

Sadly, the needles lined up along my spine by that well-meaning acupuncturist in the early 1990s had little impact. Any positive effect they might have had on my subtle energy was overwhelmed by years of cumulative illness and the hectic schedule I was keeping. No magical meridian, no unseen energy field, no pill or powder was going to save me. To heal, I had to make that plunge euphemistically called "lifestyle adjustment," the strategy that remains the number one treatment for CFIDS. I had to pare down my life and rest.[1]

Prescriptions for tonics veil the complexity of this disease, ignore its long history in my body, overlook the deductive knowledge that has been seeping into my consciousness bit by painful bit for over fifteen years. I've never thought, as many ill people say, that my body has betrayed me. I have betrayed it, by ignoring its constant rain of messages, its subtle and not-so-subtle warnings of its weaknesses and limits. The only way to dig myself out of this hole I'm floundering in is by a canny and absolute listening, putting an ear to my own chest, to what my body knows.

The atmospheric quiet and distended time of illness provide this space for listening and sifting. Illness forces not only a slower life but a slower, more meditative way of knowing. It gives room for intuition, for body knowledge, for attention to subtlety and one's own internal rhythms. The cacophony of suggestions, this influx of other people's anxieties, is a screen, a diversion. This is the first time in all my years of illness I have had the luxury to not only listen to my body but act according to what I hear. No class to teach, no conference to attend, no party to go to. If my body, heavy as if pulled by magnets, says lie down, I do. I have to. Fatigue is a self-correcting feedback loop.

The idea that if I lie in bed day after day I'm not doing enough is a curious one when you think about it. Rest is unfairly impugned. In fact, it's a highly productive state in which the body is hard at work, repairing and reprogramming. The appearance of idleness—how unjustly maligned idleness is—is deceptive. My surface languor hides a terrific inner scramble to get things working, to keep up with the demands of a body in disarray. I like Robert Louis Stevenson's famous defense of the idler: "Idleness so called, which does not consist in doing nothing, but in doing a great deal not recognized in the dogmatic formularies of the ruling class, has as good a right to state its position as industry itself."[2]

Now don't get me wrong. Many CFIDS symptoms—pain, sleep problems, depression—can and should be treated. I begin my day, as many people with CFIDS do, by counting out my pills, setting them in a blue cup on my bedside table. My vitamins, extra calcium for my bones. My herbs to turn down the voltage on hot flashes. My herbs to help me sleep. My quercetin and homeopathic remedy to dampen the sneezing fits of allergies. I confess I'm as quick to the draw as anyone to pitch a favorite remedy, proving once again that experience does little to foil human nature. I'm not immune to that automatic urge to help. I suppose illness reveals that driving force in all of us, the desire to beat back what limits, hurts, or threatens us, exposes us as vulnerable or weak or compromised.

But to heal I need much more. Writer and CFIDS sufferer Kat Duff puts it succinctly: "With a desperation familiar to many sick people, I tried all manner of diets, remedies, and visualizations, searching for a cure without success; in the process I wasted a great deal of time, energy, and money, which would have been better spent learning how to live with CFIDS, rather than attempting to escape it."[3]

I spend hours plugged into my relaxation tapes, imagining my veins running with a cool, fluid elixir of green or blue, calm and renewing. I need rest, quiet, long stretches of empty time, clouds, my noodle soup and greens, and that unfailing tonic, love. And someone to rub my hot, aching feet. The soles of my feet have become a strange barometer, a measure of the chaotic body that can't get things right, vacillating between a freezing cold that takes hours to warm or a radiating heat. The top of my head, too, sends off an astonishing heat, as if a red-hot rod runs through my body, letting off its incendiary chemical reaction in a spew of sparks at both ends. And my toes ache, every joint.

My neighbor Nancy anchors the end of the bed, cross-legged, lifts a permed strand of black-brown hair from her eyes, and takes my feet in

her hands. She, too, has been traipsing over with hopeful lists of acu-
puncturists and doctors, tinctures and salves and thick books I need to
read, especially after I asked her to sit with me one afternoon while Bill
was out. She'd picked her way with great élan through pee buckets,
wadded pajama tops, mushy tissues, and dubious salad bowls of wet
washcloths, as if she did this every day. She's a midwife, after all, with a
fine appreciation for the ragged indecencies of the body. But after that
the little lists appeared, the concerned phone calls to Bill.

This day she takes a different tack. Gently, she slides her thumbs
along each aching toe and down my arch. Her fingers trace the rough
calluses of my heels in a meditative rhythm. Like me, her hair is showing gray and she's braless under a comfortable cotton top. She slips my
feet under her shirt and places my soles next to her skin, flat against the
space between her breasts. She's hot flashing, and the bottoms of my
feet, cold at this moment, press against her chest in a cooling balm. It's
a tender, sisterly gesture. A sedating calm spreads through us both.

This is what I need. No talking, no thinking, just the feel of body
heat infusing my veins like new blood, warming me. The heat of her
body, the ice of mine, an intimate exchange of temperatures as we try to
right these careening bodies. Nancy seems content to sink with me into
a tired Buddha-trance, and it occurs to me that in our silence she is listening to me, to what my enervated body is saying: I'm too ill to talk, I
need to do nothing but rest. I need you to be silent, too, to join me in a
restful quiet. In silence, the terrible disjuncture between myself and others—the fatigued body in sharp contrast to vibrant exuberance; the misunderstandings and misconceptions—is whittled away. To be tended in
silence is to be joined. She takes deep breaths and closes her eyes.

9

Listening

What clues there are to this disorder lie presently in listening carefully to these patients. . . . Most of those from the corridors of academia
and government research offices have not listened carefully to more
than a handful, let alone the thousand or so it would take to get a feel
for this both monstrous and subtle disease.

— Dr. Paul Cheney, quoted in *Osler's Web: Inside the Labyrinth*
of the Chronic Fatigue Syndrome Epidemic

In 1816 a seemingly minor invention put a major mark on the
face, or I should say body, of medicine. That was the year the
French physician René Théophile Hyacinthe Laennec invented the
stethoscope. With this instrument in hand, physicians no longer had to
confront the unpleasant task of placing their ear against the hairy,
fevered, clammy chest of a patient, the odor of bedclothes and sweat
invading their nostrils. They could listen to the inner rattlings of disease
from a respectable distance. They could remain upright while their
patient was supine. And—once it evolved from a one-eared wooden
contraption to the two-eared instrument with rubber tubing we recognize today—they could wear this new snakelike appendage slung
around their neck as a visible reminder of their office and status.

Laennec's revolutionary discovery was inspired by modesty: one day
he was presented with a rotund young woman whose age and sex kept
him from applying his ear directly to the chest. In a flash of imaginative
association, Laennec recalled that if a person placed his ear to the end of

a wooden beam and scratched the other end with a pin—a popular drawing-room amusement—the sound came through clearly. "It occurred to me that this physical property might serve a useful purpose in the case with which I was then dealing. Taking a sheet of paper I rolled it into a very tight roll, one end of which I placed on the precordial region, whilst I put my ear to the other. I was both surprised and gratified at being able to hear the beating of the heart with much greater clearness and distinctness than I had ever before by direct application of my ear."[1]

No small invention, that. By listening to the body's noises—the raspy breath, blood gurgling in the thoracic cavity—the doctor gained clues to internal disease states that formerly could only be deduced by external signs and the patient's report of symptoms, or revealed in an autopsy. Doctors heard as never before the discordant sounds of the body, and this new listening became, like echolocation, a new kind of seeing. It was the ears, not the eyes, that sketched the inner terrain of illness, the tubercular nodes and excavations, the liquid sacs and leaks. Until the discovery of the X-ray at the end of the century opened the body to the eyes, the stethoscope was a benchmark of scientific medicine and the main tool for detecting internal disease in a living person.

As always, this low-tech breakthrough held greater implications than was first apparent. It was the inconspicuous beginning of technology as a source of medical distancing and medical hubris, the disturbing, smelly patient kept at arm's length. And it was the beginning of a shift from reliance on a patient's story of illness (now deemed subjective and unreliable) to faith in objective measures of disease. Doctors' reports were no longer filled with the patient's account of symptoms, her shortness of breath or pain in the chest or loss of appetite, but of detailed anatomical findings: "There was distinct pectoriloquism near the junction of the sternum and left clavicle."[2] Observes medical historian Roy Porter, the "sick person, gradually wasting away, has effectively disappeared, having been replaced by the patient's pleural cavity."[3]

In hospital wards filled with patients, doctors could listen over and over to the disturbing sounds of illness—"a sound resembling fluctuation, in the left side, when the patient coughed, and the metallick tinkling when she spoke"—then correlate their clinical findings with the lesions found postmortem.[4] The sounds they heard became a more trusted signal of pathogenesis than the patient's litany of complaints. Physicians were solidifying the idea that objective data determined disease. Laennec developed such a fine-tuned ear for disease that he became a renowned expert at diagnosing bronchitis, pneumonia, and tuberculosis, to which he himself ultimately succumbed, diagnosing not the same as curing. Doctors were becoming exquisite listeners—but they were listening to specific, isolated parts of the body, not the patient.

I'm as happy as any doctor not to have his ear to my chest—the relief cuts both ways—but I wonder about this instrument, and all of its high-tech offspring, that both magnify and distance the bleepings of the body. What gets listened to, what ignored?

My doctor has taken to sitting down in the small metal chair of the exam room when I go to see him, his foot flung over leg in a relaxed gesture. I once read a study that said patients feel more listened to when the doctor sits down, even if the physician doesn't actually spend more time with them. All these hard-core materialists erecting a hall of mirrors with a feint of body language. I wonder if my doctor read that study.

I'm afraid I'm jaded. Take this 2002 article in *JAMA: The Journal of the American Medical Association,* citing the rise in chronic illness that "will irreversibly alter the traditional doctor-patient relationship." Is the medical establishment finally catching on? The thought gives me a shocked rise of hope until I read further. "The new patient-physician relationship for chronic disease features informed, activated patients in partnership with their physicians," words that shine with a progressive, enlightened sheen until you notice the fine print, still shot through with medical paternalism and certainly not taking into account a misunderstood illness like CFIDS. What does this new partnership model look like? Collaborative care involves "shared expertise with active patients. Professionals are experts about the disease and patients are experts about their lives."[5]

I don't think so. I'll bet my thermometer there's no doctor at my HMO who is even remotely an expert on CFIDS, or candidiasis, or multiple chemical sensitivity. We patients, downloading the latest study on orthostatic intolerance or brain-wave abnormalities, are usually far more informed than our physicians. Once in the early 1990s I was seeing my internist, who knew I had CFIDS, for a routine checkup. This overly chipper doctor had a shiny face and permanent smile, and always struck me as a resolute booster for the joys of cheerfulness.

He was merrily palpating my breasts for lumps, chatting away, and mentioned he had just seen the musical *Cats*. "You should see it, it's great fun."

It's not easy to be assertive while lying on your back in a blue paper gown. I drew myself up with as much dignity as possible, clutching the flaps of my paper vest, and looked him in the eye. "Doctor, I'm not able to go to plays in the evening. I have CFIDS. My day is basically over by late afternoon."

"Oh," he beamed, "you look fine to me."

And this was the doctor who had been recommended as the person at my HMO who knew the most about CFIDS. Another time, so ill I could barely speak, I called the advice nurse for an appointment. "I heard it's not really an illness," she said. "What do you think?" The *advice* nurse.

No, most doctors are not experts on this illness. And we patients are not just experts about our lives, we're experts about our bodies. We know what we're feeling, what our symptom history and evolution have been, how our symptoms correlate with activity or diet, which treatments help and which don't, and much more. We have a profound level of knowledge and experience, gathered and observed over long periods of time, that a physician has no inkling of unless he or she listens to us. And it is knowledge crucial to the understanding and management of our disease.

Which is not to romanticize the voice of the body. The body can mislead or be misread. The complaints of the body can be colossally, disastrously, ignored, by patient as well as physician. I look no farther than myself.

In a repeated scenario from the early 1980s, I see myself collapsed on my maroon overstuffed couch with its saggy springs, the living room vibrating with my exhaustion. Those were the days I ran the itinerant teacher treadmill, San Francisco State University one night, Contra Costa College the next. Twice a week, after hustling my daughter off to school—Cinderella barrettes, peanut-butter sandwich and all—I plowed my way sixty miles north to a Napa Valley College satellite campus in the heart of the California wine country, gulping a high-protein drink out of a quart-sized mayonnaise jar as I left the Bay Area behind and entered the small valley towns.

In spring the days were sunny, the roadside spread with leafy rows of wire-strung vines. In a one-room prefab by the side of the highway, a dry breeze coming in the door, my creative writing students, mostly retirees, would snap open their faded blue binders or pull a crumpled manila folder from a plastic purse and spill their remarkable stories. There was ninety-year-old Russian Tanya—*white* Russian she'd always insist—barely four feet ten inches, who wrote shrewd, self-deprecating one-page vignettes. When she realized I had a sore throat one morning she disappeared without a word and returned carrying aloft a steaming cup of Lipton tea—she lived two blocks away—two sugar cubes perched on the white china saucer. And Italian Rudy, the retired police officer whose story about stopping a speeding mother whose baby's diaper was soaked through and scrambling to aid in a diaper rescue had us in stitches. Or the darkly handsome Eastern European man whose name and country-of-origin I forget, who left us speechless when, in response to a free-write exercise using the word "stone," he poured out an impassioned, wrenching prose poem about being imprisoned. I often felt less teacher than librarian, bringing up musty stories consigned to the library basement and trying to prod them back into circulation, knowing these voices would rarely be heard beyond the small circle of their origin.

At noon, exhausted, I'd bolt a tuna sandwich and head down the narrow highway to my afternoon class fifteen minutes away, cutting through eucalyptus-shaded glens, past Christian Brothers' medieval-looking stone winery, past the walled compound of Beringer's, the steep gabled roof of the German chalet just visible through languorous strands of elm. Grape-rich country air blowsed in my face. It seemed particularly galling, unseemly, to be ill amid this elegance and fecundity, to be too fatigued to poke around the gullies and wineries and byroads.

Maybe I need to exercise, I'd think, struggling to understand my enervation. Maybe I need fresh air. Maybe the vineyards with their squat sideboard houses, horse pastures, and long, straight lanes will revive me. I'd set off down the road. After ten yards that iron-dragging fatigue would press me to the ground, my head in a billowing cloud. I'd sit on a low concrete wall one block from the classroom, overtaken with the strangest sensation of a wavering lightness and heaviness at the same time, unable to go on, those undulating vines a blur.

Having hosted since 1965 the herpes simplex 1 my teenage love had bequeathed me, I knew a virus could live in the body and flare up for years on end. This exhausting illness of mine, though with very different symptoms, emulated the herpes pattern to a T: the initial outbreak hit the hardest; over time the flare-ups became gradually less severe and shorter in duration with longer periods of quiescence in between. It was an easy leap for me to assume I had some kind of recurring herpeslike virus.

When I settled onto a gray vinyl exam table one day in the ubiquitous medical cubicle with its scuffed linoleum, I suggested as much to the young intern who had bounded into the room.

"There is no such thing," he said with immense confidence. He had a wet-behind-the-ears enthusiasm that threw his body into motion. Flapping his arms and pacing the small exam room, he explained with expansive pleasure how there are hundreds of cold viruses, each one putting on a different hat, and I was catching a different one each time.

Exasperation and anger would come later. At that moment I was so taken aback and confused I couldn't respond. I had never had anyone tell me so bluntly that what I experienced in my body couldn't be happening, wasn't so. It was an initiating moment, precipitating a rather fuzzy working out of inner dissonance, in which I managed to hold conflicting notions in a loosely bound conglomerate: I had a recurring virus and there was nothing wrong with me.

I knew the doctors I saw didn't have a clue. One asked me if I could run up a flight of stairs, and when I said I could if I absolutely had to, he was satisfied that I was fine—a comment reminiscent of the dismissive attitude towards hysterics in the nineteenth century, when physicians observed that a hysteric had no problem running if there was a fire. But in my own way, I was as unsuspecting as my doctors. In my early thirties at the time, I still possessed that youthful belief in invulnerability. The concept of a serious chronic illness was not in my mental repertoire. A herpeslike virus, in particular, seemed something my body would handle, if I could just get the rest I needed. In my exhausted fantasies I was sure six months on a beach in Hawaii would take care of things; in reality I spent my evenings doing some creative math, trying to figure out how to add up my "hourly instructor" paychecks so they'd cover the rent.

I once had a heated spat with a good friend because I was, again, too fatigued to go on the hike we had planned. David, a public defender, paced the wooden floors of my flat in exasperation. He has acetylene blue eyes that shine with a religious intensity under white-blond eyebrows. He turned those eyes on me. "It's not normal to be sick all the time. I deal with murderers and crazy judges all day and I don't get sick. There's something wrong with you."

I was furious, misunderstood, in odd collusion with my ignorant doctors. "There's nothing wrong with me," I snapped back. "I'm just run-down. My blood tests are fine. You don't know what it's like to be a single mother, commuting all over, trying to make ends meet."

It was clear to me this healthy man with a decent income and no kids had no concept of what it was like to live on the edge, with no savings, no chance to stop working, even for a few weeks.

Chalk it up to the single-minded focus on survival, the folly of youthful invincibility, my surety I could plug through this and anything else life dished up. My body's clues that this illness was something more serious (rest helps but doesn't cure, these episodes are continuous, the fatigue is of another order) were intimations I heard as if on another frequency and simultaneously overrode. My conclusions were shaped by what I knew (flulike viruses are wretched but innocuous), just as my physicians' perceptions were shaped by their medical training and scientific worldview.

Listening to the body is not the instant, facile undertaking New Age promoters would have us believe. Without a larger framework of knowledge, the body's cues can be heard yet misinterpreted, the incongruities explained away or kept below the level of consciousness. Explanations are, as philosopher of science Laurence Foss has written, "framework dependent," meaning the sweep of medical vision is as confined as its premises, and we can't see what we don't know/believe exists.[6] Before the germ theory of disease and Robert Koch's identification of the tuberculosis bacillus in 1882, people believed the dank, stench-filled urban air in which they lived carried the illness. Florence Nightingale suggested TB was "induced by the foul air of houses."[7] The miasmic theory of disease, though prescientific and aroused in part by moral judgments about the lower classes and urban squalor, was partially true. Crowded, unsanitary conditions do encourage the spread of disease, though it's not the "miasma" or air per se that causes TB. They had it half right.

And so did I.

Books could be filled with stories of misreading the body; in fact, it could be argued that every reading of the body is contingent, limited, incomplete, as our knowledge and experience constantly expand. But I knew something back then that no physician was listening to. As they did with me and have done with countless others, the professional, expert classes too often dismiss this revealing body of self-knowledge as backward, uninformed, irrelevant, or inconsequential. When a normal test result is used to dismiss a person with CFIDS, this is not only an example of medical ignorance, it is a dismissal of lay knowledge, of a personal somatic wisdom. "Experience," writes sociologist Ulrich Beck, "—understood as the individual's sensory understanding of the world—is the orphan child of the scientized world."[8]

I've been fascinated to discover in recent years the emerging literature by proponents of what is called "narrative medicine," an update on the medical humanities that focuses, as its name implies, on narrative or story.[9] At the core of narrative medicine is the radical notion, rescuing us from the shoals of technological drift, that a patient's story matters and should be paid close attention. Borrowing the terminologies and strategies of literary theory, narrative medicine focuses on decoding the patient's story like a literary text. Innovative thinkers both inside and outside medicine—physicians, sociologists, humanities professors, ethicists, philosophers—use terms like "narrative competencies" to give academic cachet to the basic idea that doctors ought to know how to listen to their patient's story, and that they don't always. "It is not enough," writes literary scholar David Morris, "to declare listening a virtue, as if its value were self-evident or context-free; physicians must know *why* to listen, *how* to listen, and what to listen *for*."[10] The key here is the belief that the patient's story—the choice of words, the omissions, the metaphors, the plots and subplots—is a veritable treasure trove of clinical information.

Much has been made since the 1970s and '80s of the importance of clinical listening, and many physicians struggle to add sensitivity and bedside manner to their repertoire of medical skills. Proponents of narrative medicine aren't talking, however, about a limp attempt to add a two-hour seminar on listening skills to an unchanged medical curriculum. They're advocating a significant shift in the way medical information is gathered and digested and diagnoses are made. "Empathetic listening," according to David Morris, "that values the speaker, while crucial, is not identical with clinically effective listening which leads to accurate diagnosis."[11] In other words, narrative medicine isn't merely a touchy-feely exercise. When you increase listening skills, proponents claim, you can open new avenues of medical understanding and investigation.

Physician Rita Charon is now director of the innovative Program in Narrative Medicine at Columbia University and lectures widely on the importance of a doctor's competence "to recognize, absorb, to interpret and be moved by the stories of illness."[12] Medical interns in Dr. Charon's program and others like it read and parse literature to discern the narrative arc, the position of the speaker, or the meaning of a particular silence. They debate "intersubjectivity" and "subplot" and "discursive strategies." They're trained to approach the intricacies of listening as a practical and essential skill that will make them better physicians.

Within narrative medicine circles, there is vigorous ongoing debate about the equation between reading literature and more effective doctoring, and particularly about what kind of literature one should read. Any good novel? Only literature about illness? Only books written by those who are ill? Like many, I'm skeptical that a few good novels can stem the technological tide. Does having an overworked, coffee-drenched group of medical interns meet at eight A.M. under blinking fluorescent lights to discuss narrative voice in "The Death of Ivan Ilych" really result in more nuanced and effective listening? Does it help these interns "not lose sight of the lives out of which patients' choices come and into which medical therapy must intrude,"[13] as professor of medicine Kathryn Montgomery suggests? Does narrative medicine, as Dr. Charon and her colleagues write, "enable physicians to recognize the power and implications of what they do," help them to "better understand patients' stories of sickness and his or her own personal stake in medical practice," and "offer new perspectives on the work and the genres of medicine"?[14]

Ideally, perhaps. In reality, injecting literature into the medical curriculum in order to remind physicians of the humanity of their patients and the power of their patients' stories is, I suspect, an endeavor that succeeds when physicians are predisposed to think in humanistic terms and can sustain that intention through grueling years of work that often push one in a less sympathetic direction. Think of all the doctors whose moral sensibilities are keenly alert when discussing Hemingway's ghastly story "Indian Camp," but who nonetheless gripe with their colleagues about their "noncompliant" patients.[15] Or psychiatrist Arthur Kleinman, who argues eloquently for an ethnographic attention to the patient's story and culture in his book *The Illness Narratives,* yet still concludes that a patient, chronically ill following mononucleosis and displaying symptoms of a postinfectious illness that sound remarkably like CFIDS, was most likely suffering from depression and demoralization related to tensions in her life.[16] This is a disheartening example of the way attention to the patient's personal and social life can be twisted to reinforce a psychosomatic interpretation of disease.

Despite my skepticism, I'm all for this intersection of science and literature as a vital counterbalance to dispassionate technicality and narrow vision, and as a way to raise significant questions about the doctor/patient relationship and medical practice. To the extent that medical interns can carry into their work a greater awareness of biomedicine's subtle biases and assumptions and a greater appreciation for alternative stories of illness, patients can only gain. I particularly applaud a focus on illness memoirs, since it is in these messy, unsubdued stories of illness that the rich insights of the patient's perspective come into view.

To read an illness memoir is to inject directly into the vein. It's not round-about literary discussion. These stories present the raw realities of illness, the twenty-three hours and forty-five minutes a day that the physician, hamstrung by a fifteen-minute encounter, never sees. They remind us that there are two stories of illness, that of the patient and that of the doctor, and both deserve thoughtful attention. They remind us that medicine is an interpretive art, not always a science, and that a physician's interpretative act can have damaging as well as helpful consequences. When a doctor truly listens to the patient's narrative, the patient's story of her body's rebellions, when he or she reads memoirs of illness, a shift in perspective and care is indeed possible.

On November 20, 1975, in Lyme, Connecticut, Dr. Allen Steere, a first-year fellow in rheumatology at Yale–New Haven Medical Center, had just this faith in a patient's story when he listened to artist Polly Murray. She and her family had been suffering for years from disabling neurological symptoms, swollen joints, rashes, and fever. Some doctors thought she might have lupus. Others were sympathetic but unable to help. Many threw up their hands. After being dismissed by numerous doctors who accused her of being hypochondriac, obsessed, or depressed—some even suggested her whole family had a psychogenic problem—she finally found Dr. Steere. "He asked me to start at the beginning. Right away I was struck by his openness. He was understanding and unhurried in his approach. I didn't feel that I had to rush through sentences; here was a doctor who was ready to listen, who was genuinely interested in the story."[17]

Ms. Murray's perseverance and Dr. Steere's careful listening and curiosity, along with the interest of a number of other physicians, opened the door to the discovery of Lyme disease.[18] When I read the account of this medical mystery and its unraveling, what leaps out at me is the fact that these doctors were attentive and intrigued, and saw Ms. Murray's story as a new, potentially revealing puzzle to be solved. They were prepared to integrate the anomalous experience of the patient into their medical judgments.

Clinicians often claim that 80 percent of a diagnosis comes from listening to the patient's description of symptoms. But when doctors restore the patient's story of her illness as a valued component of medical practice, they go beyond the standard medical interview—what are your symptoms, how long have they been going on?—to draw on a broader bank of data than that normally allowed in scientific medicine. To truly listen to the patient's story is to invest the patient with authority and to be willing to hear details that challenge standard medical categories, precepts, and thinking ("I'm not just catching one cold after another"). Physicians who listen to a patient's experience, even when that experience conflicts with accepted science, practice a kind of hybrid listening, listening outside the grooves of their training while using that training to consider the medical problem before them.

When a doctor listens with a keen, open-minded attention, it isn't just the patient's words that are being restored as part of the medical dialogue, but subjectivity itself, the experiential knowledge of the patient. The physician is recognizing subjective experience as a valid part of scientific investigation, a significant element in deciphering illness and making scientific judgments. Rather than viewing the patient's account as unreliable, a source of distortion and interference, the physician sees it as a valuable resource to harness.

Is listening more than a practical and medical issue? Is it also a moral issue? Sociologist Arthur Frank writes, "Listening is hard, but it is also a fundamental moral act."[19] When we talk about ethics and medicine what comes to mind are the big questions: assisted suicide, stem-cell research, gene manipulation, cloning. But many proponents of narrative medicine see a vital link between listening and ethics, calling this juncture "narrative ethics." Drawing on the work of philosopher Stanley Cavell and ethicist Paul A. Komesaroff, David Morris calls for a "micro-ethics of the everyday," in which we investigate the small day-to-day moments typically rendered invisible, left out of the discussion.[20]

One of the primary ways we show respect or disrespect for someone is through language—whether we listen or walk away, whether we interrupt, whether we dominate conversation, whether we use words that are condescending or appreciative. So to listen is not only a way to collect and distill information from the ill person, it is a show of respect for that person. What would microethics include? Morris suggests, "It would necessarily pose different questions than a bioethics based on great events. It would ask doctors how they treat their secretaries. It would ask if they leave patients stranded for hours in waiting rooms. . . . It would ask whether a doctor listens carefully—or brushes off a complaint. . . . It would ask what words a doctor uses to describe a patient. Are they words that regard the patient as a person—an ethical and moral agent— or as a collection of organ systems?"[21]

Morris, like others, sees these smaller, "less glamorous" issues as fundamental to a discussion of ethics.[22] "Doctors who neglect to gain the skills and knowledge required for clinically effective listening—although this idea is absolutely foreign to Western medicine—are engaged in unethical medical practice."[23] Strong words. But a satisfying statement to those like me who have a visceral sense of their rightness. Certainly without an unorthodox listening, medicine can't begin to take the steps necessary to reduce the suffering of those with mischaracterized illnesses like CFIDS. Thomas Kuhn has famously asserted in *The Structure of Scientific Revolutions* that paradigm shifts are usually generated from the margins, not the center, since it is at the margins that anomalies become sufficiently visible, or audible, to force serious attention. Listening in the margins—this is what interests me. Listening to the voices that usually go unheard.

I had yet another "ah-ha" moment when I learned that the home-grown empiricism that led me to believe in the early 1980s I had a recurring herpeslike virus might not be the stuff of misguided conjecture and ignorance. One of the viruses investigated as a possible factor in CFIDS is a herpes virus discovered in 1987, HHV-6, human herpesvirus 6, so named because it's the sixth herpes virus to be isolated. Like other members of the herpes family—herpes simplex 1 and 2 or Epstein-Barr, the virus that causes mononucleosis—HHV-6 is elusive and reclusive. It has the mercurial ability to play cat and mouse with the immune system, waxing and waning for years and escaping complete eradication. And like herpes simplex and the Epstein-Barr virus, HHV-6 is ubiquitous in the population. Over 90 percent of adults show antibodies to HHV-6, and most doctors believe it to be innocuous, a microbe to which the human body has long since adapted.

Yet a number of people suspect HHV-6 may play a role in CFS, perhaps reactivating when the immune system becomes dysregulated. "If you look at all of the studies in the literature about that virus and chronic fatigue syndrome," says Dr. Anthony Komaroff, "the majority of the papers, the clear majority of the papers find that that virus is activated more often in patients with chronic fatigue syndrome. . . . You can make the argument that when [HHV-6] is reactivated in some way, when for whatever reason the immune system cannot keep it in check, that it could cause chronic inflammation of the brain."[24] Even more intriguing is that a number of researchers, including Dr. Komaroff, believe HHV-6 may play a role in multiple sclerosis (MS) as well, possibly as a trigger. The fact that MS and CFS share many clinical features makes it even more plausible that HHV-6 may be implicated in both illnesses.

10

Passing

Who says I am obliged to be what you think I am? Or what I think you think I am? Or even what I think I am but sincerely wish I weren't?
—Brooke Kroeger, *Passing: When People Can't Be Who They Are*

February 1992

I didn't keep up that itinerant teacher circuit, commuting all over the Bay Area, for more than a few years in the early 1980s. It was clear I couldn't. I started an editing business so I could work at home and keep my own schedule, seeing clients in an office a mile away. Though that meant another three years of slogging along, chasing after agents and students and writers with my card until the business was fairly well established. Hard years. I hung onto one class a semester, for U.C. Berkeley Extension, and in the late '80s, my editing business clicking along, my health began improving.

It was not to last. But beliefs run deep and hard, like sediment solidified into rock: my belief in my capacity, my ability to carry on. By 1991 my health was worsening, and this belief in myself wasn't so much challenged as mixed up, a kind of garbled inner conversation between body and self. In a few short years, I had gone from feeling well much of the time, if still worn-out, to being ill ten and a half months out of the year.

February of 1992 found me, determined to get to the bottom of things, in the office of a doctor outside my HMO who had a large practice treating CFIDS patients. He had a mixed reputation in the CFIDS community; I'd learned about him by calling around to local CFIDS support group leaders. He was said to be sometimes impatient, brash, imperious. But knowledgeable.

He ordered a complete workup, blood, stool, urine. I emptied my bowels, my bladder, my veins. On this day he scanned the computer printout of results as if perusing a menu, the tip of his nose following in an invisible line his pointed finger. Tall, Shakespearian, with dark-haired good looks, he had a tone of high command. He was my age; he'd once briefly dated a friend of mine.

"Hm, hmm." He flipped through pages. Everything, inside and out, completely normal, except—at this his eyes lit with a proprietary interest and his finger tapped the paper—I had no IgE (a class of antibodies), something he often saw in CFIDS patients. This meant little to me. But something else he said meant a lot.

He leaned his back against the wall, hands clasping the rolled-up printout behind him like a bat. I peppered him with questions about the body that were really questions about the soul, and finally asked about my chances of recovery.

"You'll always have this illness."

His words slapped me like a plunge into icy water, one that leaves you numb and tingling and shocked long after. How could he say something like that so definitively? I had always been sure I would get better, sure my years of illness would be limited. I imagined I would refer to them as "those years in the '80s when I had that virus."

I left his office rattled and angered by his cavalier words. I'd dismissed the doctors I'd seen throughout the 1980s—the ones who pronounced there was nothing wrong with me—knowing their observations about my illness were wrong. This one with his disturbing pronouncement that I was indeed ill, permanently ill, I also dismissed, unable, unwilling to believe he could be right. I didn't go back. Some years later I learned he'd left his medical practice and gone to film school.

It had been more than a decade since I had crossed the line into chronic illness and encountered physician disbelief and ignorance, bio-medical limitations and biases. Now I was crossing another border, entering another new world, one that would require a changing self-image, a wrestling with meaning, and a confrontation with cultural atti-tudes and interpretations of illness, with stigma and otherness. I wasn't yet ready for this crossing.

I wanted that exhausted self behind me. I had believed in the late 1980s, as my health improved, that I was discarding that ill self. I rebelled at the thought that she could once again take up residence, become a part of me. On a downhill slide, I faced the difficult, convo-luted challenge. Who am I now? Do I continue the story I'd so fervent-ly believed—I'm just run-down, I'll get better—now that I knew I'd invented it all along, albeit out of ignorance? This belief in ordinariness, so avidly held against the complaints of the body, how could I now give it up? Especially since much of the time my illness allowed me to appear to function normally, why should I relinquish the privileges of anonymity?

As someone raised with that ramrod-straight Protestant ethic of self-reliance, that training in stoic perseverance, I found the idea of "coming out" as a seriously ill person hard to swallow. All evidence to the contrary, I believed I could get better, believed I could soldier on with only small, private adjustments. The truth about my body I held at arm's length, like a disturbing object I could neither let go nor accept. That "run-down" story, ruse that I now knew it to be, allowed me to cling to what I had. I stuck with it.

I went on with what I was doing, focused on other things, the things that mattered. I met my writing clients, showed up for brunches and par-ties, heading for a comfortable couch to ease my aching muscles, sitting mutely if I was too exhausted to talk. One hostess thought I was rude because I didn't jump up to help with the dishes. Other people who didn't know me well simply concluded I was the quiet type. The misconceptions grated, but they seemed better than the alternative. "Avoiding disclosure," writes sociologist Kathy Charmaz in her book on chronic illness, *Good Days, Bad Days,* "allows claiming other identities than illness."[1] Passing, to all except those closest to me, enabled me to pull a protective cloak around something vital in myself, some key element of identity. As long as I had an invisible illness, people met me as simply the person I was, writing consultant, teacher, neighbor, not as an ill person.

Throughout that spring of 1992, in the tall-windowed rooms of Dwinelle Hall on the U.C. Berkeley campus, my fiction students and I debated the uses of the unreliable narrator and interior monologue, a breeze carrying in the monastic noontime bell of the campanile. But the washed-out undercurrent of my illness was there. Only one week that term did I feel well enough to teach. The other nine weeks I went through the motions as if underwater, dredging up thoughts through a thick viscosity, my voice launched against the weight pressing my breastbone.

When I browsed through my student evaluations at the end of the semester I came across one that sent a hot singe through my chest. "She seems low energy." Instead of mailing it in with the others to my administrator, I threw it away, something I never did, even when I got a bad write-up from the occasional grumpy student who rated my class slightly above spoiled fish. That comment—she's low energy—was a crack in my story, a tear in a screen. I didn't want it seen. I would rather have someone disparage my teaching than disclose my secret self. It pains me now to think how unspeakable those words were to me, how hard I worked to prevent their utterance. Those words stung not only because they exposed my illness. They revealed that all my efforts, all my performances, my willingness to continually hurl my ill self into the world, all that was not enough. This illness was becoming stronger than all my impersonations, all my willpower.

How is resistance expressed when the body is ill? By controlling the narrative, what you choose to reveal. By ensuring that other people's view conforms to the one you want to be true. By investing others with the normalcy story, making them the carriers of the picture of reality you can no longer maintain within yourself. If they don't see the truth, you can feel saved. The liberation achieved when others don't see is a false liberation, but it's a way to protect a self under siege. This deliberate deception, Kathy Charmaz suggests, "may also provide a time buffer during which a person can begin to adapt to change."[2]

I remember the jarring moment a friend referred to me as disabled, probably in 1993. Sprawled around my living room, a group of woman friends and I were trading midlife hormone horror stories. Marcy, who has a disabling back injury, was lying on her back on the carpet in an old baseball jacket and mentioned something about being disabled, then waved her hand vaguely in my direction. "Oh, Dorothy's disabled, too." Her words shook me. I'd never thought of myself as disabled, never would have attached that word to myself. Was I? Ill, yes. Exhausted, yes. But disabled? I slid the word around in my head for months after that, knowing on some level it fit. In some ways, in some contexts, I was.

When I asked Marcy how she handled the situation of working with a disability, she said she told people of her limits or special needs on a need-to-know basis. But my friend Myrna, a lesbian, said to me gently one day as I expressed to her my angst about "coming out," "It's always best to be fully who you are." I wasn't so sure. To come out as a lesbian is a matter of identity and pride. You want to value and embrace who you are, so others can as well. But do I want to embrace an identity as an ill person? What does it mean to incorporate into one's identity physical limits, pain, and incapacity? What alchemy could transform the body's shifting, unseeable complaints into a positive sense of who I am? I had a deep ambivalence about identifying with this part of myself, about letting it define me.

In the face of certain, irrevocable disability, like becoming suddenly paraplegic, you're forced to adjust and take on a new identity. Author Reynolds Price, faced with paralysis after treatment for a spinal tumor, advises those in a similar position not to try to continue being the person they were, but to become "someone else, the next viable you."[3] A paraplegic may feel a phantom, shadowy former self still there, may struggle to reconcile old and new, but he or she daily confronts the unchangeable, concrete reality of a radically altered self.

With an invisible illness and gradual decline, nothing is so clear. You can remain for years in a borderland of confused identity. When things are not black-and-white, but marbled and shifting, how and when do you accept an identity as an ill person? Where is that clear-cut point of delineation, a line you cross, a specific moment you say, there's a new me here I have to acknowledge? Was it last month? This week?

One day in the summer of 1993 I dialed the number of a CFIDS support group, an act that in itself was a capitulation. I'm not sure what impelled me, whether it was a voyeuristic curiosity or some inner instinct that I was descending to a place where help and connection would be vital. Did I really want to hear others lament their brain fog and fatigue? Did I want that mirror lifted up to me—this is what you are, this is where you fit in? I was holding myself apart with the snobbery of the able-bodied, even though most of the time I could no longer place myself in their company.

A woman from the group gave me directions and explained the elaborate carpool arrangements they had devised to make travel easier. "I drive to the BART station and meet Charles, then I lie down in the backseat while he drives over to Linda's. Then Linda drives the rest of the way there so Charles and I can rest."

She offered to hook me into their driving loop. "I can drive myself," I said tersely.

We met in a young man's sparse, depressing apartment, one of those square, cinder-block places students call home. This felt increasingly like a wrongheaded venture, going backward in time. A circle of hard, mismatched chairs. Cracked, random tea cups. All nice people. Very nice. A bearded young man unable to work who lived with his mother. Huddled under an afghan, a ponytailed newly married woman—the one I'd spoken to on the phone—disabled by a flea-fogger her husband set off two days after the wedding. A petite, curly-haired speech therapist with all the appropriate therapeutic language, how we need to open a space for healing. And on the futon couch a feverish man slick with sweat, half-lying, half-sitting as if just pulled from a river, a shiny leather jacket tugged around him. He was profoundly depressed and suicidal.

My bones ached in the hard wooden chair. Exhaustion poured through me. I needed to leave.

"I don't think I can go on." His voice wavered up from some deep pool of despair.

The ponytailed woman reached her afghan over him. The speech therapist went into high gear about healing spaces.

How do you excuse yourself when a group of people you've just met are trying to talk someone out of suicide? Well, good luck, I have to go now. What I'd hoped would be an experience of patient empowerment was fast becoming a sinkhole. The disabled trying to save the drowning.

Guilt-ridden, I stayed longer than I should have. I didn't go back.

Passing is something you do when you're alone with an inner world, and it's something that makes you more alone. Yet it's an attempt to be less alone, to blend in, to fit a public notion of what the self should be, what is valued and rewarded. In my own stumbling way in the early 1990s—going to a doctor, a support group—I was trying to be less alone, to find support and understanding, others to lean against, someone to spread an afghan over my tired limbs. But to be truly less alone you have to loosen your grip on the determination to blend in. You have to face what it is that marks you as different.

"Spoiled identities" is what sociologist Erving Goffman called it: the identity that doesn't conform to a society's ideal, that carries stigma, otherness, shame. "An individual who might have been received easily in ordinary social intercourse possesses a trait that can obtrude itself upon attention and turn those of us whom he meets away from him, breaking the claim that his other attributes have on us."[4] These words strike me with a sharp clarity. Just as often as an ill person is met with compassion, she is met with judgment. Something about the state of being ill—the vulnerability, feebleness, sign of weakness or defect—invites opinion and inference, or at least wariness.

Although today there is a growing disability pride movement, it hasn't permeated the culture or changed public attitudes in the way the gay pride movement has. There is still an enormous stigma attached to the wayward, uncontrollable, sometimes offensive, imperfect body. And there are hierarchies of stigma; some conditions carry greater disgrace than others. Someone who has no control of his movements or who drools will be more ostracized than an otherwise healthy paraplegic. These hierarchies are internalized even by those who are ill.

Poet J. D. McClatchy offers a revealing comment about his good friend, poet James Merrill. Everyone knew Merrill was gay and knew, as his health declined in the 1990s, that he was ill. But he kept secret the knowledge he had AIDS. Says McClatchy: "For once, he had had difficulty speaking about something; his lifelong frankness about his homosexuality never yielded to an ability to talk about the still more volatile subject of his AIDS. It was the only situation in which I've found him literally speechless. . . . But it's in the nature of this disease that the accounts of its onset are shrouded in repression, lies, half-truths, forgotten circumstances, etc."[5]

Like a stain, the taint of AIDS—its unsavory implication of sexual

transgression and licentiousness, of bodily fluids and orifices—adheres
to its victims. Those with CFIDS are also defiled. Our transgression,
unexplained fatigue, is less egregious, less reviled, but still condemned.
The stigma of illness carries a particular tinge, reminding us of our bodily failings, from which—unlike race/ethnicity or sexual orientation,
other stigmatized identities—no one is immune.

It's this pervasive fear of the body's frailty that creates the palpable
stigma of illness. In a society like ours that places high value on productivity and effort, on energy and vigor, the weakened body is deeply suspect, and feared. The weakened body that doesn't recover is even more
suspicious. You must not want to heal. You must have given up hope.
People leap in with antidotes and suggestions. I'm referred to the Center
for Attitudinal Healing, or offered Caroline Myss's book, *Why People
Don't Heal,* offers loaded with presumptions.

Like Philoctetes, Sophocles' character who has a wound that will not
heal, the chronically ill become the "other," stigmatized and isolated
because of their unreasonable bodies. One of Sophocles' late plays,
Philoctetes is that rare literary record of raw, agonized physical pain, and
is much-quoted by those who write of illness. I had to order a copy
when I kept coming across references to it. Paging through the slender
paperback, I found myself enthralled and appalled by this over-the-top,
groveling, desperate, miserable character. His story is not what we might
expect from Greek drama, and as critic Edmund Wilson has pointed out
in his acclaimed essay, "Philoctetes: The Wound and the Bow," it is not
one of Sophocles' popular plays.[6] There is no temple or palace, no love
angle, no heroic and cataclysmic battle. This is a tale of a wounded warrior, a fallen hero, alone in a cave, writhing in anguish and shrieking in
pain. Philoctetes' great battle is with the ravages of his own body, with
the pain of desertion, with betrayal.

As with so many illness narratives, Philoctetes' tale is that of a journey waylaid: on his way to Troy with the Greeks, Philoctetes is bitten by

a water snake at the shrine of the goddess Chryse. Instead of healing, his wound becomes ulcerated and putrid, marking him with a constant, undeniable sign of his otherness. The wound is so odious, his shrieks so unbearable, his companions cannot bear to be around him. They abandon him on the island of Lemnos for ten years and come back for him only when they need his magic bow to win the Trojan War.

Here he is as he rages and laments his betrayal by his fellow Greeks: "This is where they abandoned me, alone with my wound. . . . Can you imagine what it was like for me, waking up here after they'd gone? Getting up that day? Imagine the tears, the cries of anguish. Picture me, seeing the ships I had travelled with all gone and not a soul here: no one to help me; no one to ease the weariness of my affliction."[7]

The flawed, wounded body in this story is repugnant and repelling. It transforms Philoctetes from warrior to outcast, confined to an island and left to survive on his own wits. He is exiled to his own territory, where the polluting effect of his wound cannot contaminate others, much as lepers inhabited their "cities of the damned" or the insane their asylums, which originally meant sanctuary. Sanctuaries become prisons.

Philoctetes suffers from his wound; he suffers more deeply from isolation. Aristotle's very definition of what it is to be human is based on social connection: a being who is part of a social structure, a *polis*. This, he said, is what separates man from beast. Isolated and abandoned, Philoctetes descends to bestial conditions, living, if it can be called that, in a harsh cave, wrapped in foul rags, shivering in the chill wind.

Those who are disabled will say—and I know what they mean— that it is not the disability (wound, flaw, illness) that is the greatest burden and source of grief. It is the reaction of others that is most devastating, the barriers erected through stigma, misunderstanding, rejection. Behind my fear of identification with the ill is the ultimate fear: that like Philoctetes I will be left behind. Left to a small, circumscribed world. Deprived of the company of the healthy, who will sail away.

But there's more to the story. Philoctetes has a terrible wound, but also a mighty strength. His magic bow, a gift from the god Heracles, doesn't miss its mark. His ability to wound others, a kind of contagion, gives him a deadly power, a power the Greeks need to win the Trojan War. He is, as Edmund Wilson writes, both "wounded and indispensable."[8] But is he indispensable because of his superhuman strength or because we can never successfully abolish the wounded from our company?

Perhaps what is so magnetic and essential about Philoctetes, what keeps readers coming back to him, is neither his wound nor his bow, but his double nature. This doubleness, as both wounded and wounder, rather than setting him apart, reflects what binds us. Sophocles seems to be holding up Philoctetes—his raw agony, his godlike strength—as a powerful and fearsome mirror, in which we view ourselves in all our bravery and dissolution, in which we see our potency and our vulnerability to pain and suffering. Philoctetes knows this vulnerability: "See how frightening and precarious mortal life is—one moment all is fine, the next it's not."[9]

In Philoctetes we see the capacity we all have to crumple, to rage and lament our fate, and the capacity we have to rise above what befalls us. In his fellow Greeks, we see our capacity to reject the frail, and the necessity of retrieving the wounded into the social body. We can deny frailty, leave behind those who suffer, but it won't work. Eventually, we have to go back for them. We can no more banish the ill from our society than we can avoid or ignore our own wounding. We must face down our fears and denial of illness, weakness, and suffering, in others and in ourselves. Ultimately, we must see that the "other" is ourself.

We may feel apprehensive about an affiliation with the ill or disabled, about coming face-to-face with suffering. Yet through alliance we develop understanding and compassion. And compassion is what will deliver us from our own suffering, as the oracle at the end of *Philoctetes* declares: Philoctetes will be cured of his wound when he forgives the Greeks for abandoning him and uses his magic bow to help win the Trojan War.[10]

I sometimes think of that drowning, suicidal man at the support group, hugging his arms around his leather jacket, his face slack with despair, and wonder what happened to him. Did he get better? Worse? Is he still sweating through his sickness? He seemed almost unreachable in his island of misery. And I had backed away, fast, to save myself from a similar drowning.

"Why didn't you tell me what was going on?" a colleague and friend, Susan P., asked me years later. She was miffed that I'd kept from her the facts of my illness, that I hadn't let her help. I flailed about for an answer. To tell someone who knows me I'm ill is to deliver a punch line, a surprise, eliciting a radical transformation of her perception of who I am and requiring she go through, in a small way, the same process of revision I have. There'd been times, out to dinner or at a meeting with other writers, my head fat with exhaustion, when I'd formed the words in my mind, ready to spill them. Something always held me back. It's amazing how strong is the grasp, as to a lifeboat, on that old self.

Was my silence akin to the denial of the alcoholic, or the resoluteness of the person who doesn't want to face impending decline? Was it projecting a fictitious self, or keeping an old self from leaving me? Was it independence taken to the level of folly? Or fear of what might lie ahead? Or shame, that skulking partner of weakness? Or avoidance of the projections and misconceptions of others, always close on the heels of the ill, especially with an illness so little understood, so open to misinterpretation, as CFIDS?

I could paint it many ways. I only know that I was packing my body each day into sweaters and bright scarves—a crucial accessory for the pale-faced ill—the way a teenager crams herself into pants one size too small out of an intense need to have them fit. It was what I needed to do. As long as I could get away with it, I would. In the end it was my body that spoke, no longer able to keep up my double life. It was my body that brought an end to my time of passing.

11

Protean Phantasmagoria

It's always been said that this is an illness of exclusion, that everything else must be ruled out before the diagnosis of chronic fatigue syndrome can be made. This is not true. The pattern of symptoms is unique; there is no other illness in general medical practice that looks like this one.

—Dr. David Bell, quoted in *The CFIDS Chronicle*

March 1996

When I'm not cursing my body I'm vaguely amused by the imagination of this bug I have, its sly power to shift and mutate and surprise, my body the playing field for an attention-grabbing, phantasmagoric exercise. As I worsened in the early 1990s my litany of symptoms expanded, and since my crash in 1995 the list has assumed encyclopedic proportions, from light and sound sensitivity to nausea, through sleep problems, night sweats, muscle weakness, and more kinds of pain than anyone would care to hear. In a cruel game of addition, each symptom seems to find a new ecological niche in the fluctuating ecosystem of my body. At times I feel little more than a vessel to a parasitic colony busily building its infrastructure, planning future expansion with an industry and fervor I can't begin to match.

This mid-March morning, Saturday, yet another new symptom catches me by surprise. I'm listening to paper rustlings and zippers and book thuds from Bill's office as he packs his bags for Central America, under pressure to complete work for a MacArthur grant to study and write about democratization in Nicaragua and El Salvador. He's taken a leave from lawyering and is stuffing short-sleeved shirts, spiral note-books, tape recorder, laptop, books and more books into his suitcase. His timing is impeccable, some instinctual mechanism telling him it's time to get out of town. I'm weaker than usual, as if some giant hand were pressing my body down. When the airport van arrives I'm starting to worry, but I figure I'll feel better after lunch.

Bill gives me a parting pep talk, stooping in front of the bedroom chair I'm slumped in and patting my knees. "You'll be fine."

"I'll be fine."

He's off.

As the day wears on, I can tell I'm sinking. A stabbing pain spreads through my muscles, ibuprofen no help. Lisa is at Raleigh's hoisting beer mugs, working the evening shift. I call my neighbor Pat and ask her to come down, just to have someone in the house. She watches TV down-stairs until I'm ready for sleep. A soothing presence.

Sunday morning I'm worse. Something is hitting me hard, a light-ning-sharp, pinching pain all over my body, tiny snaps of electrical charge, stronger in my extremities. A rush of new anxiety. After fifteen years, I thought I knew this illness, its surges and retreats, strategies and patterns. But its capacity to transform, its wild inventiveness, throws me off guard. I leave a message for the doctor outside my HMO who has a large practice treating CFIDS patients and whom I've seen several times. A few hours later his partner is on the phone. He knows little about CFIDS.

"Could be magnesium deficiency. Your electrolytes could be off. If it gets worse you should go to the emergency room."

I'll do anything to avoid that netherworld of fluorescent lights, hard plastic chairs, and vacant, catastrophe-ridden waiting. I send Lisa to the store for Gatorade and toss down vitamins. The pain is taking my breath away.

Lisa, as frightened as I, helps me into a warm bath. She cranks up the heat until the small room is incubator-warm, then hunkers down on the toilet seat. She looks harried and uncertain.

I crouch in the steamy water, knees to chest, my body gangly and strange. The hard bottom of the tub hurts my bones. My calves hang like loose, lifeless hammocks. How fast the body deteriorates, leaves behind robust form and becomes something else. I have no words for what I'm experiencing, what is going on in my body, this disintegration from the inside out, like fruit that browns and softens to the pit.

Lisa shifts on the toilet seat, one leg crossed over the other. Hot air chugs through the vent in the ceiling.

I'm embarrassed to be so infantile, so naked, to have my daughter bathing me like this, to be so frightened. The heat is making me woozy. "I hate this, I hate this. If only I knew what was going on."

I run a finger down my bony shin. I'm baggy and loose and skinny as an old woman. I've lost five pounds, down to 105. My sit-bones hit the ceramic tub like junkyard metal. Light as I am, even a tub full of water doesn't buoy me. It would take much more to lift me from this tonnage in every limb.

"What I would like to experience most of all," wrote Primo Levi, a Holocaust survivor who carried the terrible weight of memory, "would be to find myself freed, even if only for a moment, from the weight of my body."[1] He never did experience that freedom, not in life, anyway. He died from an apparently suicidal fall down his apartment stairwell.

"Don't stress, Mom. Try to think about something else. Try to just relax." Heading up crisis central is not Lisa's idea of how to spend a weekend. She doesn't know what to do, and neither do I. We sit in silence, a liquid gurgling coming up from the drain.

When Levi thinks of lightness his mind conjures astronauts, "as much at ease as fish in water."[2] As if a new medium—air, water—can bring a metamorphosis out of pain, shedding some earthly, burdened status. Strangely, the atrophy of my sedentary body is similar to that produced by weightlessness. The muscles smaller, bones thinner. This makes no sense to me. To be heavy as a tank and wasting away at the same time.

"Can I rub your back?"

"Gently." Lisa's small hands press into the skin of my neck, fingertips running down the slope of shoulder. Her touch is tentative but practiced, a dancer's touch, necks and muscles her territory. But even the slightest pressure hurts, as if I'm bruised all over.

She hands me a towel. I heave myself upstairs, faint and wavery with heat, and sink like a stone into bed.

Later, Lisa brings a plate of white beans and cherry tomatoes, rich in magnesium, the sliced, glistening tomato halves ringing the plate in an ordered, aesthetic design. She sets it on my bedside table with a flourish, her face transparently hopeful, an expression that chokes me up. A circle of tomatoes to ward off our chaos.

First thing Monday morning I call for an appointment with my internist. Frazzled, Lisa loads me in the car and steers me through the sliding doors of the hospital in a wheelchair.

When I describe my symptoms, my doctor, a kindhearted but clueless Asian man, wants to know if I'm hyperventilating. He makes me breathe into a brown bag. "Is that the same feeling?"

"No!" I practically shout, though I can barely talk. I'm furious at his trivializing, and demand that he order blood tests to check my electrolytes and magnesium levels.

But already the symptoms are backgrounding into something more familiar. By that evening I can tell I've caught a cold; Lisa, who gets colds constantly, has had one the last few days. The virus has triggered in my deranged body a deranged response, as if my nerve endings are frayed, ragged cord, my central nervous system shorting out. Over the next two months, crackling and receding, the pain works through its cycles, sometimes tolerable, the prickle of a foot asleep, sometimes so metal-sharp I lie on my back in tears.

Even weirder, at the end of the two months, in what feels like a last frenzied assault before subsiding, my symptoms migrate in such rapid succession as to defy credulity. One day I have intense brain fog, tight pressure in my head, confusion, headache. The next day my head eases but my biceps are "attacked," becoming so painful and weak I can't use my left arm at all. The next day my arm is better but my chest feels foggy and weighted. I imagine my body as the feeding ground for a colony of high-speed migrants that constantly move on to new territory for better grazing.

Physicians familiar with CFIDS often refer to its protean, migratory nature, its symptoms that wax, wane, transfigure, reappear. Not only do symptoms shift within patients, but among patients with CFIDS some will have more trouble with confusion and brain fog, others with chronic sore throats, others with vertigo and dizziness.[3] The basic outlines of this illness are consistent—overwhelming fatigue, a brain that doesn't work, a body that hurts—but the individual expression carries a curious, unique stamp.[4]

Bill comes home to this new calamity. (Though the flare-up triggered by my cold peters out after two months, the needle pinches, that bed-of-nails yogic torture, will continue to wax and wane, gradually declining over the next two years.) Rather than being revived by his time away, he seems depressed by what greets him, the sick-ward bedroom and washed-out partner. My setback unnerves him and dredges up renewed despair. He's got another trip to Nicaragua planned for June. I can see the worry playing through his mind, visions of me worsening, of him not being able to go.

Wooden and remote, he carries in my soup, exchanges my cold washcloth for one steaming hot. Emotionally he's dead, spent. His eyes don't meet mine, his body is contracted against everything around him.

When he sits for a moment at the end of the bed, remote control in hand, to flick on the news, I lean over and put my arm around his shoulders. He doesn't move, doesn't turn his head, his eyes beaded on the TV.

I feel abandoned at the time I most need his love and encouragement, and this floods me with red-hot fury, a shot of adrenaline up the spine that has me tossing and twitching at night, my mind plotting escape. I'll get my sister Martha who lives forty-five minutes away to come get me. She would, at the drop of a hat. All my sisters would take me in an instant if I asked, they're that way. Ill as I am, I have options. I plan what I'll pack, how I can get things together. . . .

But in morning light, anger deflated, I realize my folly. The battle of needs, this flailing after survival, this flood of inexpressible emotion that threatens to swamp us, seems to shrink and pale. A calmer rhythm prevails. We get through another day, and another.

"I'm getting stronger every month, even with this setback. Can't you see?" We're lying in bed.

Bill looks doubtful.

"Oh ye of little faith." I give his shoulder a shake, trying to buoy the man I need to buoy me.

He rallies, brings me a special plate of black beans and red peppers from the deli. At night, we curl on our sides and I warm my cold feet against his calves. All sorts of thoughts, remnants, pesterings, careen around in my head like fireflies in a jar. There they'll stay. My sore throat, which had just begun to ease, is back with a vengeance. I've been shut back in my silence, bringing a new despair, like being sent to prison for another sentence.

Explanations. How we flounder through the wilderness of confusion searching for explanations, those words that can orient our world, lay it out like an undisputed map. A friend who's been bedridden with a CFIDS-like illness—no one knows for sure—for two years and undergone every test imaginable, from muscle biopsies to thyroid tests, says if only someone could explain what was going on, then she could relax. A common sentiment, the need to know, to understand, to battle back the wilderness of fear, to bring from chaos, cosmos, a world of understandable, manageable outlines.

If the confusing multiplicity of CFIDS symptoms is the patient's undoing, it is the medical profession's despair. Scientific medicine has trouble with profusion, with patients who have too many symptoms, those so-called "thick-folder" patients. I read of one woman with CFIDS who was told by a physician there was nothing wrong with her when she complained of severe stomach pains. Several months later she was diagnosed with advanced colon cancer. After treatment, she confronted the dismissive physician: "'I don't know if it was because I was a woman or a lesbian, but at some time you stopped listening to me.'... 'I don't think it was because of those things,' he said, 'but it was because of this,' and he held up my thick medical folder.... 'You had too many complaints.'"[5]

Such untenable excess has led doctors to dismiss whole battalions of patients. French psychiatrist Jean-Martin Charcot had a name for the multitudes of neurasthenics who showed up at La Salpetriere in the late 1800s. "*L'homme du petit papier*" he called them, these patients who appeared grasping little slips of paper on which they listed their endless array of symptoms—"*petit*" certainly tongue-in-cheek.[6] The image strikes me with a kind of grim humor: I imagine the little lists crumpled, misspelled, repetitive, disordered; crib notes for the exhausted neurasthenic mind unable to remember the details of its own distress, and mirror of its disarray—except I know it's really an image of desperation. Illness as inventory. A monologue of the body held out to the doctor for interpretation. Make sense of this! Decipher this chaos.

The question of CFS's lineage doesn't disappear with neurasthenia. By the early twentieth century, neurasthenia had faded into psychogenic territory, but clusters of fatiguing illnesses that appeared similar to neurasthenia continued to be documented in the United States and Western Europe well into the twentieth century. Though disputed, a physical explanation as to their origins prevailed. The listing of these epidemics—L.A. County in 1934; Punta Gorda, Florida, in 1956; Royal Free Hospital in London in 1955, among others—reads like a roster of unfamiliar names on an old genealogical chart. Are we related? Can we find in the outlines of these epidemics an obscure prehistory to CFIDS?

It's unclear. Little research, medical interest, or follow-up accompanied these outbreaks. Anthropologist Norma Ware notes that following the discrediting of neurasthenia, "chronic fatigue had become invisible," given "no name, no known etiology, no case illustrations or clinical accounts in the medical textbook, no ongoing research activity—nothing to relate it to current medical knowledge."[7] But if you trace the lineage, you can uncover several little-known stories of inquisitive epidemiologists whose findings are strangely resonant with descriptions of CFIDS today. One such story is that of Donald Henderson.

In May of 1956, a Florida state epidemiologist had requested that the U.S. Public Health Service's Communicable Disease Center in Atlanta (what was to become the Centers for Disease Control) send officers to take a look at a puzzling outbreak of illness in the small town of Punta Gorda. Donald Henderson, chief of the Epidemic Intelligence Service, sent EIS officer David Poskanzer to investigate. When Poskanzer returned to Atlanta to make his report, he emphasized the curious nature of the symptoms he observed. Henderson later recalled how Poskanzer kept insisting, "They were protean, absolutely protean."[8]

After Poskanzer's initial visit, Henderson himself traveled to Punta Gorda with a small team. Through community interviews they identified among the 2,500 residents 62 cases in addition to the 30 already diagnosed. Eventually, they would record 150 cases.[9] Henderson saw firsthand the protean symptoms Poskanzer had described, documenting a long list of complaints: fatigue, headache, neck and muscle pain, confusion and memory impairment, muscle weakness, vertigo, depression, anxiety. The investigators also noted a higher incidence among women, medical personnel, and those between the ages of twenty and fifty; the absence of deaths; and the "curiously prolonged and relapsing course."[10]

Henderson and his team eventually concluded that "mass conversion reaction" was unlikely, and that the patterns of the illness were "consistent with a hypothesis of person-to-person transmission of an infectious agent," though they could never isolate a particular microorganism.[11] They summarized their findings in a 1957 article in the *New England Journal of Medicine,* and, acknowledging a history of various names for similar syndromes, chose to call the illness "epidemic neuromyasthenia."[12]

Henderson later said, "Epidemic neuromyasthenia is a most ungrateful disease. . . . Its manifestations are subjective rather than objective. . . . There was practically nothing that we could see or touch or measure. I mean, there were no lesions to examine, no big livers or tender spleens to feel, no jaundice, no classically paralyzed limbs, no laboratory data to analyze. We used to sit in my room at the motel after dinner and puzzle it over and over. None of us had ever seen anything like it. We just couldn't put it together."[13]

Reading Henderson's words makes me sit up and take note. When you've been wandering alone in the realm of illness, these hints of possible companionship are arresting. Perhaps there are answers here, or at least clues, a direction to investigate. Which is just what another investigator thought. Enter Alexis Shelokov.

In the same issue of the *New England Journal of Medicine* in which Henderson and Poskanzer reported their Punta Gorda findings, an epidemiologist named Alexis Shelokov wrote an account of a puzzling disease he had documented among fifty student nurses at a psychiatric hospital in Rockville, Maryland, in 1953 that was originally thought to be polio.[14] A polio expert, Shelokov didn't believe what he was seeing was poliomyelitis. Curious, he began searching the medical literature for reports of other outbreaks that had an odd flavor, "any polio epidemic that didn't smell right,"[15] and found himself poring over a detailed eighty-five-page report by epidemiologist Sandy Gilliam about an outbreak of what Gilliam called "atypical polio" in L.A. in 1934.[16]

In May of 1934, as what appeared to be a virulent polio season got under way, a rash of health-care workers at the L.A. County Hospital began taking sick. Polio patients were flooding hospitals; over 1,700 cases would be reported in the L.A. area by July.[17] In this fear-laden atmosphere, the health workers were assumed to have contracted polio. They were quickly isolated and given serum therapy. Only later would the odd facts emerge: what was going on that summer was much milder than was typical of polio. A report about that year's epidemic published in 1937 in the *Bulletin of the Los Angeles Neurological Society* noted the "scarcity of the usual."[18]

The epidemic that year, though widespread, resulted in fewer deaths and almost no paralysis. Of the 198 health-care workers who took sick, most did not have spinal fluid abnormalities and showed transient paresis (muscle weakness) rather than paralysis. It was also unusual to have such a high percentage of young and middle-aged adults affected by an illness that more often targeted children.

The National Institutes of Health had sent A. G. "Sandy" Gilliam to investigate, and though he was struck by the unusual profile of that year's cases, he nonetheless viewed the polio virus as the culprit. After the L.A. County outbreak subsided, the nurses sued the hospital for compensation. The settlement stipulated that no one discuss the case, and as a result, there was no follow-up on the affected health-care workers. Dr. Byron Hyde, a Canadian physician and researcher, later learned that "many of the staff doctors never returned to full employment."[19]

Although none died, many of the 198 affected workers continued to have debilitating symptoms for years.[20]

The Punta Gorda and L.A. County outbreaks are not the only ones that hint at an intriguing link with CFIDS. In the medical literature are accounts of other enigmatic epidemics, often named after the place they occurred: Icelandic disease, an illness that developed in 1948 among over one thousand residents of Akureyri, Iceland, and was originally suspected to be polio; Royal Free disease, in which three hundred people, mainly staff members of the Royal Free Hospital in London, took ill in 1955, also initially confused with polio; an outbreak in 1936 affecting thirty-two of sixty-three members of a convent in Fond du Lac, Wisconsin.[21] These epidemics and others like them shared familiar features: flulike onset with low-grade fever, headache, sore throat, and malaise, followed by months and years of continuing mental and physical fatigue, muscle pain, and mood and sleep disturbances. In all of these cases no pathogen was isolated, though investigators generally felt an infectious organism was to blame, and there were no mortalities.

No one name ever emerged to describe these illness clusters. They were variously called Icelandic disease, benign myalgic encephalomyelitis, epidemic vegetative neuritis, epidemic neuromyasthenia, atypical poliomyelitis, and a number of other terms. After a 1956 editorial in the *Lancet* used the term "benign myalgic encephalomyelitis," that name gained wider currency: "benign" because no one died, "myalgic" to indicate muscle pain, and "encephalomyelitis" to indicate central nervous system involvement. Significantly, the names benign myalgic encephalomyelitis and epidemic neuromyasthenia were based on patients' descriptions of their symptoms—which suggested problems with the central nervous system and muscles—rather than laboratory findings.[22] Forty years later, advances in technology had made researchers more confident that their instruments could reveal any existing pathology.

Now, the lab would trump the clinic: very similar symptoms and incapacities would be labeled "chronic fatigue syndrome," because there was no "solid evidence" of muscle weakness or brain and spinal cord inflammation.[23]

Were all these illnesses linked? In 1959, Henderson and Shelokov published an article in the *New England Journal of Medicine* addressing the 1934 L.A. epidemic and twenty-two other similar outbreaks that had erupted between 1934 and 1958, noting "the apparent similarity in the courses of illness, the common nature of most symptoms and signs, the remarkable paucity of abnormal laboratory determinations and the similar epidemiologic characteristics."[24] In their concluding article published a week later, they asserted, "It is probable that further epidemics will occur," and recommended using the name "epidemic neuromyasthenia" "until an etiologic agent or agents are identified or until the underlying pathophysiologic processes are defined."[25] The terms epidemic neuromyasthenia and benign myalgic encephalomyelitis continued to be used to describe sporadic outbreaks of persistent fatigue in the 1950s and '60s.[26] Interestingly, in a 2004 interview at his home, Donald Henderson said that the Punta Gorda, Florida, and Rockville, Maryland, outbreaks "were, in effect, what we now call chronic fatigue syndrome."[27]

So why wasn't CFIDS more readily seen as aligned with this medical history? Why should its array of symptoms have been excuse for dismissal and denigration? Curious, I put the question of these prior epidemics to three physicians who were among the first to treat patients with CFS and who took this illness seriously from the beginning. Dr. Anthony Komaroff had seen patients with a lingering flulike illness in his general medicine clinic in Boston in the late 1970s and, his interest aroused, had led the investigation of the Tahoe epidemic in the mid-'80s. His words are telling, bringing to light a black hole of medical knowledge. "If I put myself back into the early 1980s, at that point I had never heard of epidemic neuromyasthenia, and virtually none of my colleagues had ever heard of it. If you went into the literature you could find it, but ... it was perceived as a rare, unusual event and you can't possibly cover everything in the course of medical education."[28]

When I speak with Dr. David Bell, who treated a large cluster of people with CFS in his Lyndonville, New York, practice in the mid-1980s, he echoes these sentiments. "Nobody had ever heard of it. I'd never heard of it until about 1988. I'd studied [CFS] for three years before I ever heard about any of these earlier epidemics.... [They were] assumed to be a minor detail related to polio."[29] I ask him if he thinks chronic fatigue syndrome is the same as these earlier outbreaks. "Oh yes," he replies quickly, "no doubt about it."[30]

In the San Francisco Bay Area, internist Carol Jessop was another physician who began seeing patients with a persistent flulike illness in 1984. That year, in the process of doing research into the mysterious ailment, she came across descriptions of these prior illness clusters. "I remember writing grants and referring to those epidemics and that we thought we were having another one. But I don't know if it got out into the general [public]."[31] On September 30, 1987, the *San Francisco Chronicle* ran an article about what was then called chronic Epstein-Barr virus (CEBV), and listed these earlier epidemics. But such references were isolated and unusual. Though a few physicians who saw large numbers of CFS patients began putting the picture together by the mid- or late 1980s, most practitioners and the general public had no awareness of the historical record.

Dr. Komaroff adds, "We now know, from the epidemiologic studies that Harvard did in the 1990s and the CDC has done, we now know that a condition that meets the criteria for chronic fatigue syndrome is more common than we would have imagined twenty years ago, than doctors would have imagined. But back in the early 1980s there wasn't a single study that was even under way, let alone published, that tried to determine how frequent an apparent postinfectious fatiguing illness might be in the community at large."[32]

In fact, even when the CDC finally conducted prevalence studies in the early 1990s, the investigators used flawed epidemiology, resulting in a gross underestimate of the disease prevalence—remember those CDC figures of 3,000 to 10,000 people in the United States with CFIDS that patient groups so heatedly disputed? The CDC had relied on physician referrals to identify patients—a method that misses all those people who don't have a physician, whose physician fails to recognize their illness, or who are too ill to get to a doctor—rather than a community-based survey. When Leonard Jason and his colleagues used a community-based method in their study of a Chicago suburb published in 1999, the numbers leapt to a frightening 422 per 100,000, or approximately 836,000 adults in the United States with CFS.[33]

There's yet another mystery here. Even if physicians weren't familiar with these prior epidemics, why weren't they aware that a virus or pathogen of some sort could have a chronic aftermath? How could this viral behavior remain such a well-kept secret? Since I'd walked around with recurrent herpes blisters on my mouth for fifteen years before I came down with CFIDS, I'd always been baffled when physicians I saw in the early 1980s balked at the idea of a persistent viral infection. Dr. Komaroff's comment on this point came as a surprise to me, revealing an astonishing gap between medical orthodoxy and lived experience.

"When I graduated medical school in the late 1960s," he explained, "and for the next decade, viral diseases were thought of as temporary illnesses. Either they killed a person, which was rare, or the person's immune system finally routed them, after a struggle and a period of illness. Sometimes the virus caused permanent damage, and sometimes not. But the virus was ultimately eliminated from the body. That was the belief. . . . When I first began lecturing about CFS in the late 1980s, most doctors in the audience, who had been trained decades earlier, did not think of viral infections as capable of causing long-term infection and relapsing illness."[34]

It turns out I—who have never been in the forefront of anything in my life—and thousands of others have had the misfortune to be in the first wave of an epidemic that would defy prevailing medical wisdom about viral infections, and whose earlier incarnations were buried in the dusty archives of medical history. Also, it's hard to recognize a complex illness like CFIDS for what it is when it appears in scattered rather than epidemic form, as was the case in the late 1970s and early '80s.[35] What all this doesn't explain or excuse, of course, is why so many providers dismissed or denigrated those of us with CFIDS for the first twenty years of this current outbreak.

Here is a speculation of my own: With the corrective of time, medical historians will line up the earlier epidemics of myalgic encephalomyelitis and neuromyasthenia with CFIDS, using the wide-angle vision not available to the individual clinician of the 1980s who had an overflow of patients in the morning, a noon meeting he was late for, and to whom the symptoms of a CFIDS patient easily resembled psychoneurotic or ubiquitous complaints. But even the corrective lens of twenty years of experience with this illness doesn't erase a core question: Shouldn't doctors have been more curious? If you're confronted with patients who don't fit the medical mold you've been taught, shouldn't this pique your interest? Lead you to page through a few medical history books? Cause you to wonder, to reflect with an open mind? Some doctors do, but precious few. Yes, there is sometimes a blurry area between psychosomatic complaints and these confusing illnesses. Yes, professional pressures within the medical and scientific community discourage maverick thinking or deviation from accepted medical views. Reputations are at stake, sometimes economic interests or loyalty to a sponsor. But still.

"I think that in general physicians find it very frustrating if they don't get an easy answer to something," Dr. Jessop reflects. "I think they're taught in Western medicine that all symptoms relate to some kind of functional syndrome or disease state that they have read about in a book. And when things don't line up and they don't get an answer, in Western medicine, especially during the earlier periods, the '70s and '80s, it was just, well, it's in their [patients'] head. That was it.

"What the medical community I hope has learned is that there are a lot of things that happen to patients that we don't understand, and that we're still uncovering the mysteries of the brain and the immune system and how they function, and that when patients come to us and say they're having problems with fatigue or brain functioning, or they just can't do the kinds of things they used to do, we need to be open-minded."[36]

Drs. David A. Shaywitz and Dennis A. Ausiello in a 2000 *New York Times* article, "The Demise of Reflective Doctoring," describe how the recent focus on efficiency and speed has altered medical education. They cite several studies that show a decline in a physician's ability to conduct a basic physical exam. But beyond the fact that medical encounters are now more cursory and impersonal, and perhaps less competent, Shaywitz and Ausiello assert that something even more vital is being lost in the name of efficiency: the time to reflect about individual patients, to think creatively and expansively about clinical experience. "This matters because medicine is more than simply the compassionate (and now, efficient) application of received wisdom; it is also the challenging of old customs, and the development of new insights. It is critical to recognize that an academic clinician is both a provider, whose goal is to assimilate and then thoughtfully apply a given set of information, and a medical scientist who questions traditional dogma. . . . We must encourage doctors in training to ask fresh, penetrating questions, to wonder about underlying biological mechanisms, to consider alternative therapeutic approaches."[37] The result of this neglect, this lack of original, innovative thinking, is the delegitimization of illnesses like CFIDS.

Dr. Bell muses, "I just regret that so many people have been hurt so badly, and it was never necessary. If doctors were just doing what they were supposed to do, which is listening to patients, taking their complaints seriously and offering compassion and the best that they could do in symptomatic treatment, people would be much better off."[38]

Is CFIDS nothing more than a confusing array of variable and mercurial symptoms? Or has the conventional medical lens obscured a clearer view? Those clinicians and researchers who have studied this illness extensively and seen scores of patients have observed over and over the coherence of CFIDS symptoms. They point to the lack of an adequate clinical case definition in the United States as the real source of confusion. In Canada in 2003, a group of physicians and researchers compiled a clinical working case definition to "encourage a consideration of the ongoing interrelationships of each patient's symptoms and their coherence into a syndrome of related symptoms sharing a complex pathogenesis rather than presenting a 'laundry list' of seemingly unrelated symptoms."[39]

The Canadian definition establishes four categories of symptoms: postexertional malaise and/or fatigue, sleep dysfunction, pain, and neurological/cognitive manifestations. By making postexertional malaise and neurological symptoms central to the diagnosis, the definition selects a more restricted group of patients who are less likely to have psychiatric reasons for their fatigue. As compared to the current U.S. Fukuda definition, the Canadian criteria select "cases with less psychiatric co-morbidity, more physical functional impairment, and more fatigue/weakness, neuropsychiatric, and neurological symptoms."[40]

Yet in the United States, since 1988 patient care has been guided by case definitions that have been acknowledged as inadequate. First the

1988 Holmes definition, then the revised 1994 Fukuda definition of CFS—both research definitions, not clinical definitions—focused on fatigue rather than on the cardinal symptoms of postexertional malaise, brain and sleep dysfunction, and pain. The CDC is currently working to revise the Fukuda definition, but for the last two decades physicians have lacked an effective tool to help them understand and diagnose patients.

Reading the four categories of the Canadian definition, I feel a gratifying recognition. Yes, these are precisely the symptoms I experience in my body. These four categories capture the sweep and contours of this illness as I know it. With this definition, the anarchic, baffling symptoms become understandable, if not adequately explained. They can, in fact, be deciphered, the illusion of chaos dispelled.

12

Brain Drain

If you think of the brain as being like a battery, it's as if the battery is being drained of power.

—Myra Preston, quoted in *The CFIDS Chronicle*

November 1996

The time of chronic illness has a quality of its own, fluid, uncalibrated, felt rather than measured. Minutes can extend to agonizing lengths. Weeks and months sweep by in a haze. "Pain—has an Element of Blank—/" wrote Emily Dickinson. "It cannot recollect/ When it begun—or if there were/ A time when it was not."

I track the rhombus of skylight-flung light that scans the carpet each day, again the next. This is my sense of time, a passing of light and seasons. Afternoons, I lay my yoga pad in this puddle of warmth and settle into it as into a bath, in gray sweats and long-sleeved T-shirt. As the flat edge of light inches along, I slide my pad with it. The sun has a medicinal capacity to quiet my aches, and at these moments I find a lulled peacefulness. Days meld, time is reduced to getting up for toast and lying back down and up again for soup. Time loses its urgency, its workday, efficient meaning. Dates and hours become an artificial concept concocted by a feverish world I'm no longer part of. Thursday? Friday? The eighteenth? Twenty-second? I couldn't say.

"Immersion time," sociologist Kathy Charmaz calls it, when illness is no longer an interruption or intrusion but a new way of life. "Like a fan, drifting time unfolds and expands during a serious immersion in illness," writes Charmaz, capturing this altered reality.[1] After crisis come the submerged, amorphous days, when the past is remote, the future vague. I've dropped into a break in time, a chasm that is as isolate and inert as an underground bunker, or a candlelight vigil, or a suspended hammock, or all of these rolled into one.

I think this sense of suspension, letting myself drift through hours of anesthetized calm, is key to healing. In fact, that most knocked out state of all, the coma, is apparently the most healing state possible.[2] And I suspect it's the vague alarm that I might descend into just such an irreversible, semivegetative state that makes me haul myself up each day to do what I can, to prove to myself that my body can still function in some semiuseful way.

So the day comes in November of 1996 when I wake feeling ready to slip behind the wheel of my old white Toyota with the gray panel on the driver's side from a cheap repair job. This desire has been needling its way to the surface for a while. I want to drive, to see if I can. I still have my fantasies. This winter I'll start driving. Next spring I'll begin seeing a few clients. I haven't driven in fourteen months, since my last limping trip to the office before my infamous New York trip, my last client, a half hour I could barely get through. I shudder to think of it.

The fall air has a diffuse whiteness to it, cloud haze and horizon merging. It smells of cold and fog, like it's come off a lake. Drifts of shriveled leaves, muted yellows and reds.

Bill comes with me, a bit grim around the mouth, but hopeful.

"Just to the office to get my mail," I say. "Maybe I can start doing it myself." Bill has been getting my mail for me.

It's strange to be behind the wheel, my right hand finding its automatic place on the smooth gear handle, right foot feeling for the gas pedal. My worry is that I won't be strong enough, won't have the strength to turn the wheel, my arms will tire, or my thighs will be too weak to stiffen against the brake and hold.

The Toyota hasn't been washed. Pine needles pile on the wipers and plaster the windshield. No water in the window spritzer. Bill sticks his arm around the window jamb and swipes at the long brown needles.

With a turn of the key the Toyota chokes into its low rumble and we're off, pulling away from the curb and putt-putting through the side streets like ordinary people. The feel of driving comes back to me in that natural, kinesthetic way that riding a bicycle or playing the piano does, with only a slightly odd sensation of something new and old at the same time, sitting in this low bucket seat with brushed gray upholstery. This is great! Through the Berkeley neighborhoods, brown shingles shoulder to shoulder with old two-story stucco bungalows, rickety slat fences, and small arching porches.

Within a few blocks it hits me. There's a crew-cut bicyclist to my right, a yellow-shirted pedestrian tugging her terrier in the crosswalk, another woman grasping the wrist of her fidgety child bundled in a pink parka on the curb. A blue Pontiac to my right, a stack of cars ahead, more behind, a red light, a green light, a stop sign. I have to keep track of all of them, and remember whether to press gas or brake, whether to turn right or left. Onto Shattuck Avenue and into the business district and there's more commotion. Delivery trucks and billboards and storefronts. Stone Mountain Fabrics, office for rent.

I pull up in the metered parking in front of my office, a narrow wooden building with a Western-style false front, sandwiched between an electronics store and billiard parlor. Bill runs in to grab my mail, and I swerve into traffic for another mile back home. By the time I'm at Telegraph and Dwight, halfway back, it's clear. I shouldn't be doing this. My brain is fuzzy and I'm squinting over the wheel, a running, frazzled dialogue in my head. Stop sign, press brake, no pedestrians, press gas, watch left.

I turn into the driveway relieved and chastened. I did it, but I won't be doing it again for a while. It's too soon.

It's not my muscles. It's my brain.

I should have known. I still can't tolerate speed, multiple conversations, simultaneous happenings. Details skim away like a hat on the wind. I write February when it's October, February when it's April, October in August. This morning I was sitting on the bed paying bills. In order to get things right, I had to stop, focus, concentrate—where am I? What am I doing? What day and month is it?—as if a patient guide had to get my attention and call me to my task. I'm in my bedroom. I'm going to write a check. This is my checkbook. I have a pen. The month is November.

Do things that involve more than one step? Forget it. When I finished I stood and surveyed the three piles of paper—waste paper, paid bills, receipts—repeating in my mind each step of what I had to do, the thoughts an overwhelming jumble I struggled to sort. Take these bills downstairs to my home office and put stamps on them. Throw out the waste paper, file the receipts, and pick up a magazine I want to read. Put the paid bills in the mailbox. Go to the kitchen and fill my water thermos. I ended up with a stamp in my hand, the thermos left in the kitchen, the magazine forgotten.

With a brain this deranged, a body so weak, I cling to what I have. Astonishingly, what I still have is my analytic mind. Moments after I've forgotten the magazine I wanted to retrieve, as if I've leapt into that miraculous phone booth and bounded out, cape flying, as a different person, I'm settled in my sunny upstairs bedroom in the curved-beech-wood chair penning comments to a writing client, critiquing his novel. "Fremont disappears too early in the story. He's a mysterious, intriguing character whose brief appearance hints at more to come. I wouldn't let

him drop out of sight so soon." My work is painstaking, only an hour or
two a day. But the words, the ideas emerge clear and cogent.

I'm amazed I can work at all, amazed at the vast, confounding intelligence of the floundering brain, that three-pound mass of slippery gray
meat, neurovasculature, and chemicals. Berkeley, California, neuropsychologist Sheila Bastien, who has tested cognitive function in CFIDS
patients, says these patients are often more impaired than those with
concussions, hypothyroid conditions, or even brain tumors.[3] She
describes people with CFIDS as having "intellectual scatter" or "pockets
of dysfunction in the brain. It would be like if I were a ninety-word-per-
minute typist but I had trouble dialing the phone."[4] Her analogy is
evocative of neurologist Oliver Sacks's description, in *The Man Who
Mistook His Wife for a Hat,* of the music professor who had severe visual agnosia: "How could he, on the one hand, mistake his wife for a hat
and, on the other, function as apparently he still did, as a teacher at the
Music School?"[5]

Dr. Anthony Komaroff has commented on the "focality of the
deficit" in CFIDS patients, "impairment of visual processing with
preservation of verbal processing, for instance."[6] This makes sense to
me. Working on the computer or driving—using my eyes to absorb a lot
of light and activity—exhausts me quickly. But I can lie on my back in
bed, eyes closed, and hold a brief phone consultation with a client with
only a few fumblings for words that go mostly unnoticed. I have to shut
out every distraction, marshal every ounce of energy to pull those
thoughts from the recesses of my brain—an urgently focused, consuming task that makes my forehead ache—but my mind zips along, analyzing, questioning, linking one thought to another in what is, to me, an
astonishing verbal display. My lips and tongue form the right words,
they're sent along the phone line to my client's ear, and he says, "Ah-ha."
He would find it hard to believe I become confused if I try to lock the

front door, put on my sunglasses, and remember to put my keys in my pocket at the same time.

These flashes of lucidity and normal functioning are thrilling. In these moments I am given back my self. Exultant, I poke my head into Bill's office, next to our bedroom, to report how well the consultation went. To feel that my analytic mind hasn't deserted me, that I still have ownership of that key component of my work life, is elating. I revel in the proof with all the joy of someone who wakes after an accident and discovers with euphoria that she can wiggle her toes, move her head and arms, recognize her family, talk.

My delight is about more than just verbal capacity. On some level it's about retaining a recognizable self. To me, the most unsettling, visceral experience of CFIDS is to feel that the self is so physically, neuronally constructed, so subject to viral invasion, disruption, distortion, so concrete and vulnerable, rather than mysterious and sustainable and somehow beyond the merely corporeal. "For we consider ourselves," Oliver Sacks writes, "and rightly, 'free'—at least, determined by the most complex human and ethical considerations rather than by the vicissitudes of our neural functions, or nervous systems."[7] Lying in a gelatinous, wobbly CFIDS haze, I can easily feel CFIDS as an assault on the basic construction of self. I skate regularly into that borderland where self and illness collide, overlap, shade one another, where the fear of dispossession lies.

What does it mean that I have to work so hard to conjure my guide, that self that knows where I am and what I'm about? Without her, I slip into confusion. The self in this state is an attenuated self. Confused, distracted, having trouble focusing, yes. But it's more than agraphia, aphasia, dyscalculia, agnosia—all those names neurologists come up with that sound like a Latin nursery rhyme, those abstract words that speak of loss, deficit, defect. My dissociation is more than an impairment of function or competence. If the sense of self is grounded in knowing who and where you are and what you're about, this basic grasp of self is challenged by neural confusion.

It isn't just a matter of a "me" that has slipped away, taken a hiatus from meaning and comprehension and action. There is also the matter of the "not me" that has taken up residence in the altered ecology of my nervous system. This "not me" is teary and labile and weak and distracted. She can't speak up, can't calmly assert herself and her needs. She cries at corny commercials, cringes at loud noises. Who is this person who needs to be driven places, who can barely coordinate the task of paying her bills, dependent and deranged?

I read in a newsletter for those with CFIDS one sufferer's suggestion for negotiating the task of cooking: place a timer next to each pot on the stove, set it for when the food will be done, then get some blankets and pillows and lie down on the floor in front of the stove. She emphasized the importance of a timer for each pot. One timer was not enough. At first I found myself laughing at the absurdity of having to take such measures. Then I thought of how many pots of food I'd burned after forgetting I'd put something on, and how often I felt I couldn't drag myself to the stove one more time to check on what was cooking, and realized this was a really good idea. With CFIDS, you laugh and cry at the same time.

"I'm still me," said Christopher Reeve after his catastrophic, paralyzing accident. "I'm still here," said Ram Dass after a stroke left him partially paralyzed and fumbling for words. In illness we exist most profoundly in our body and most profoundly despite our body. I remember standing by the bed in those early days of terrible illness, Bill at my side. He must have been helping me to the bathroom. "I'm not my illness," I insisted. When the self is most threatened it is also the most mobilized. In the face of my weakness and confusion, my difficulty concentrating, fumbling for words, I could feel a central, constitutive part of myself demanding to be recognized.

I could joke about CFIDS being the ultimate postmodern experience, that of a continuously reconstructed, unstable self. There's nothing like a postmodern experience to make a romanticist of you. Give me a stable, unitive self any day. "When we discover what we are made of," writes neuroscientist Antonio Damasio in *The Feeling of What Happens,* "and how we are put together, we discover a ceaseless process of building up and tearing down, and we realize that life is at the mercy of that never-ending process. Like the sand castles on the beaches of our childhood, it can be washed away. It is astonishing that we have a sense of self at all, that we have—that most of us have, some of us have—some continuity of structure and function that constitutes identity, some stable traits of behavior we call a personality."[8]

I've felt chastened, as ill people do, by how vulnerable the self is to its neurotransmitters and hormones. Thankfully, for me this humbleness is eased by the revelation that this same biochemical mechanism—guided by what, the unanswered question—is a potent force for health. As Oliver Sacks writes, "For the powers of survival, of the will to survive, and to survive as a unique inalienable individual, are, absolutely, the strongest in our being: stronger than any impulses, stronger than disease."[9]

The research that attempts to explain this split and disoriented self has been slowly emerging—rather like my mind these days—since the late 1980s. The medical articles are tucked away in archives or stacks of magazines in a cluttered office, or they float in the expanse of cyberspace. They get pulled into my hands as a sheaf of papers, stapled, darkly reprinted, circulated, shared, or stuck in a manila folder on my desk. These paragraphs of medical code, arcane and to me only slightly penetrable, are themselves shorthand encapsulations of weeks, months, years of messy research—calling someone for subject referrals, writing a grant, rushing to the post office, meeting with assistants while gulping bitter coffee from a Styrofoam cup. "MR abnormalities consisted of foci of T2-bright signal in the periventricular and subcortical white matter and in the centrum semiovale."

These dense pages hint at explanation, insight, understanding— other peoples' minds working to decode our own. They're probing a part of our body—our brain—not easily examined or penetrated, not easily seen. We study the brain's abilities through neuropsychological testing (e.g., can you count backward from one hundred by sevens). We peer at the brain through neuroimaging techniques—MRI, SPECT, PET—but what is revealed remains partial and inconclusive, rather like our view of CFIDS.

The picture that is developing is both illuminating and validating for me and other CFIDS patients. According to Dr. Anthony Komaroff, "Several objective biological abnormalities have been found significantly more often in patients with the syndrome than in the comparison groups. The evidence indicates pathology of the central nervous system and immune system."[10] Eighty-five percent of CFS patients report disabling cognitive problems: difficulty with memory, concentration, attention, learning, or complex information processing; slowed processing speed; susceptibility to interference.[11] Though much more research needs to be done, the existing studies of neurocognitive impairment in chronic fatigue syndrome suggest that underlying structural changes in the brain correlate with symptoms.

Remember those UBOs—unidentified bright objects—those punctate lesions that show up on MRIs of CFIDS patients, hauntingly enigmatic? Though there has been variability in findings among studies due to differences in research methods, three MRI studies considered to be relatively well constructed reveal that compared to controls, CFS patients show significantly more of these T2 signal hyperintensities in the subcortical white matter, often in the frontal lobes.[12]

Are these abnormalities linked in a significant way to the physical impairments CFS patients report? Another study by neuropsychologist

Gudren Lange, Ph.D., at the University of Medicine and Dentistry of New Jersey makes this link: "CFS patients with MRI brain abnormalities report being more physically impaired than those patients without brain abnormalities." In fact, Dr. Lange and her colleagues go on to suggest that brain abnormalities in CFS are "as functionally significant as has been shown in the case of multiple sclerosis."[13] Further studies are needed to determine if this link between CFS symptoms and MRI abnormalities is indeed significant, but the authors believe their work shows that CFS has a basis in brain pathology.

Those puzzling UBOs are not the only physical evidence of brain damage. Several studies using SPECT (single-photon emission computed tomography) scanning, which measures cerebral blood flow, have revealed a pathological decrease of blood flow in several regions, including the cerebrum, midbrain, and brainstem.[14] In another study, the authors correlated decreased frontal blood flow with cognitive impairment, and suggested that these blood flow abnormalities may play a role in CFIDS patients' decreased physical and mental functioning.[15]

In an intriguing study, researchers from American University and the National Institutes of Health have found CFS patients do poorly compared to healthy adults when asked to multitask.[16] When CFS patients had to identify letters on a computer screen while listening to random words on headphones, they performed poorly. Yet they scored normally on tests for intelligence, memory, and language. Researchers speculate this may be why CFS patients show normal intelligence but have trouble locking a door and talking at the same time. I remember once trying to write a check as Bill was saying something to me. His voice rattled in the air. I couldn't absorb anything he said. I had to put down my pen and checkbook, look directly at him, and concentrate on what he was saying to be able to respond.

Does this sound similar to attention deficit disorder? More than a few patients, myself included, have wondered about these similarities.

Once a CFIDS activist told me, laughingly, of a meeting with other persons with CFIDS (PWCs). "We were like a roomful of ADD kids. One person says, 'Oh, the lights are too bright.' Another says, 'Can you talk more slowly?' Another keeps saying, 'What? What? Could you say that again?'"

Pediatrician Michael J. Goldberg, director of the Neuroimmune Dysfunction Syndrome Medical Advisory Board and Research Institute in Tarzana, California, has studied immune dysregulation and neurocognitive disorders since the 1980s and believes CFS may exist on a continuum with ADHD (attention deficit/hyperactivity disorder) and autism. He and other researchers have found remarkable overlap in the findings on SPECT scans between adults with CFS and children with attention deficit processing disorders.[17] Dr. Goldberg believes an autoimmune/viral process may be behind these conditions.

Myra Preston, Ph.D., who owns and operates Silber Imaging in North Carolina, has used BEAM (brain electrical activity mapping) scans to reveal abnormal brain mapping in people with CFIDS, "a lack of appropriate shifting of the brain through all of the brain frequencies" that may contribute to cognitive problems.[18] She has found that people with CFIDS attempt to solve cognitive tasks with slow-wave (theta and delta) activity, while most people use fast-wave (beta) states. "It's like trying to work when your brain says 'sleep,'" she says, and suggests these brain-wave problems are similar to those of patients with closed head injuries and hepatic encephalopathy.[19] Dr. Preston found brain patterns in CFS patients that differentiated them from depressed patients, and other studies have also concluded that symptoms of cognitive impairment cannot be explained by depression.[20]

Of course, the vocabulary of the brain's malfunctions is only one part of the medical discourse on CFIDS, which involves multiple body systems. Many different investigations have identified abnormalities in the immune system, which may be involved in a reciprocal cycle of influence with the central nervous system. One hypothesis is that chronic immune activation disrupts the central nervous system, producing the symptoms patients report. Studies have revealed increased activation of CD8+ cytotoxic T cells and decreased functioning of natural killer cells.[21]

Both European and U.S. investigative teams have reported another immunological abnormality, increased levels of RNase-L, part of an antiviral pathway that is activated more often in patients with chronic fatigue syndrome compared to controls.[22] Immunologist and biochemist Robert Suhadolnik and colleagues of Temple University, the American group, subsequently documented a novel low-weight form of RNase-L in patients with CFS, a finding that could provide a biomarker for CFS.[23] The European group compared patients with CFS to healthy controls, patients with fibromyalgia, and patients with major depression, and found a higher ratio of the novel low-weight form of RNase-L to the normal 80 kDa protein in 72 percent of CFS patients compared to 1 percent of controls, a difference Dr. Anthony Komaroff calls "striking and highly significant."[24] These findings are consistent with the hypothesis that chronic infection, from either a reactivated latent virus or some other agent, leads to ongoing low-level warfare between virus and host, releasing cytokines and producing the symptoms of CFS.

Neuroendocrine dysfunction includes a down-regulation of the hypothalamic-pituitary-adrenal (HPA) axis, which produces a mild hypocortisolism that can increase immune activation.[25] Many of the symptoms people with CFS experience, including fatigue, myalgia, and sleep disturbances, are found in people with adrenal insufficiency, also suggesting an endocrine component in CFS.

Pediatrician Peter Rowe and associates at Johns Hopkins University, and others, have documented significant autonomic dysfunction, primarily orthostatic intolerance and neurally mediated hypotension, as seen on a tilt table test.[26] Since the center for control of blood pressure and heartbeat is in the limbic system of the brain, these findings suggest a central nervous system defect as a factor in CFS.

There's no question that a preliminary picture of the biological basis for CFS is taking shape. Says Dr. Komaroff, "If you take all of the studies that have been published and count up all of the patients in all of those studies, you're dealing with a pretty large number of patients and you're dealing for the most part with consistent findings."[27] Yet much more needs to be done. Besides the lack of funding, research has been hampered by methodological problems, including the small subject numbers in many studies; inconsistency in use of the case definition; reliance on a patient's self-reporting of symptoms (i.e., the patient is simply asked if he or she feels better now as opposed to a year or two or three ago, a vague and subjective measure); the lack of "staging criteria" to subgroup patients according to age at onset, length of illness, severity of symptoms, etc. (if a virus is active in early stages of the illness but latent in later stages, for instance, this can make a big difference in testing outcomes); variable lab and testing protocols and procedures; and no consensus on how to judge clinical improvement.

And there are other problems: researchers often work within their own disciplines, precluding broader collaboration; there are few longitudinal studies that gather information over a long period of time; the sickest patients, those unable to travel to a clinic, are not included in most studies—to name a few.[28]

The bits and pieces of research pile up like parts of a jigsaw, presenting an incomplete but suggestive view. These studies don't yet carry indisputable authority. At times, they seem to me to be paltry stabs at understanding and elucidation—the nineteen patients given a brief battery of questions, a quick MRI on a minuscule budget. Still, it is through this growing body of research that the illness will be made comprehensible, and through research that we will develop treatments and a cure.

Medical language, it's been said, flattens and erases the lived complexity, the uniqueness, of each individual illness. It makes illness generic, impersonal, reducing it to notations on a chart. But given the influence exerted by biomedical science, medical language also gives authority, shape, realness. It assuages skeptical minds and brings our suffering into relief, makes it apparent. So that's it. Or part of it. Maybe.

With neuroimaging and other studies, our bodies begin their emergence from invisibility. These snapshots act as an overlay to the ill body that transforms the way it is seen. These studies form the beginnings of a dialogue between the suffering patient and science, the beginnings of a shared vocabulary. "MR abnormalities consisted of foci of T2-bright signal in the periventricular and subcortical white matter and in the centrum semiovale." Thought about this way, the coded research messages seem a kind of poetry, a compressed, stenographic communiqué, like Emily Dickinson's cryptic poems that reveal a private world, rich with meaning.

The Necessity of Beauty

Everybody needs beauty as well as bread.

—John Muir, *The Yosemite*

January 8, 1997

The call comes Wednesday afternoon. I'm in that lulled, amnesiac time of day when a kind of contentment overgrows complaint, and greet my sister Alice, in Santa Barbara, cheerfully, though an edgy thought slips beneath my words that it's odd she should call in the afternoon.

She's cautious. "How are you doing?"

I blather something about having had friends over the previous weekend, doing better.

"I'm glad you've been with friends." Her voice, flat with forced calm, sets off a tremor of apprehension. I can tell something's wrong.

She drags in a breath. "Mom's in the hospital," and then the details as my hand flies to my mouth and I wrench myself up in bed. Mom and Otto separated a few months ago; she lives by herself not far from Alice. A neighbor, after not seeing her for a few days and noticing the newspapers piled up, went to check. Mom never locked her doors. The neighbor found her unconscious on the blue tiles of the bathroom floor, one arm twisted beneath her. The paramedics came, she's at Cottage Hospital—the image of a cottage flits through my mind in an oddly comforting way, though I know this is the hospital where her mother, my grandmother, died over forty years ago. She's suffering hypothermia and they're warming her.

I stumble into Bill's office, crying. He leaps up from his computer chair and grasps me around the shoulders, shocked.

A flurry of phone calls. My other three sisters are hurrying to Santa Barbara, as are my Mom's two sisters. There's no question about my making the six-hour drive, let alone flying. Travel is way out of reach. I'm still recovering from having spent two hours with friends in my own living room three days ago. Before sleep that night I cling to the doctor's words: it could just be a slip and fall. I hang onto the thought that they'll revive her and she'll be awake in the morning. I keep thinking they're warming her, that she's in a cottage being warmed.

In the morning my sister Laura's voice from the hospital slides into that ominous high pitch. "I'm sorry, sis. . . ." They've taken an MRI. Not good. Mom's brain is flooded with blood, a cerebral aneurysm.

With a sickening sweep, the ghastly realization overtakes me. I gasp and sink to the couch. Something irreversible has happened, something that can't be undone. Thoughts swamp me, of Mom as a bed-bound invalid, maimed, her face contorted, or worse. Still, I cling to hope. She could be OK. A long rehabilitation, but OK. Laura will call after the doctor comes by this morning.

Bill stays with me till noon, then has to leave. I wait by the phone, wandering around the living room, picking up a vase and setting it down, watching cars pass, distracted and disoriented. No call. At two P.M. I try the hospital.

Alice answers, her words chillingly matter-of-fact. No hope. My sisters, aunts, and uncles are all clustered around Mom's bed, singing and praying. "Amazing Grace," "Ave Maria." A conversational blur bleeds through in the background, subdued, churchlike. Martha's voice, "Do two." Alice's again close to my ear.

"There's nothing to do. We're going to take her off the breathing tube."

Disbelief hits me like a shot of ice water to the gut. "No you can't!"

I shout. "You can't give up! Why didn't you call me?" I'm shaking with helplessness, soaked in fury that they'd give up so easily, that no one called for my opinion, that the decision has been made without me.

Uncle Gordon takes the phone, my tall, sweet uncle who gave me away at my wedding twenty-six years earlier. "Sweetie, it's what's best. We're all here with her."

The spiraling race of events seems to collapse inside me. I'm devastated, sobbing. At four P.M. she dies, my family reciting "The 23rd Psalm" and watching her skin take on the pallor of death.

That night she comes to sit on the side of my bed, a gray, transparent, anguished figure, twisting toward me, arms outstretched in a desperate, despairing reach for me, for life. The next night and the next, as I sink into the vague, drifting place before sleep, these fleeting apparitions appear, like a flash card in my mind: the cowled figure of death, its face a black void, an emptiness; the faint rower in a misty boat, back turned, pulling away. I'm wrung through, in an altered, unreal state, floating somewhere above the life around me. All day I clutch the phone to my ear, my anchor, to talk (thank God I can talk!) and sob with my family. On Sunday they hook me up by phone to her memorial service at First Christian Church on Chapala Street in Santa Barbara. Bill and I huddle side by side in hardback cane chairs in my tiny home office, the only room with a speaker phone, listening to the service bundled in coats against the January chill, staring at my books and files.

Grief, sorrow, these are strange enough states, ballooning with unreality. Grief from a distance is stranger still, though space no longer matters, death having obliterated any sense of near or far. You can't be any farther from someone, nor any closer, than in the immediate aftermath of death, those distorted days and nights that shred any former assurance of physical place, of me here, her there.

Each night for the next two weeks, in the twilight of near sleep, as if breaking through from another realm, she visits, her form fading into abstract images of an ocean wave, a single rose, or a seated Buddha. These fleeting visions, thrown like flowers to my heart, are precious to me and deeply healing, in the way that connection and beauty are heal-ing. In my distraught hole of grief, these images comfort and console. I know she's come to be with me since I couldn't go to her, and that I'm with her as she leaves us.

The thought that she has vanished, that I couldn't see her as she died, and that I will never again visit her in her home, haunts me. The out-there world has already disappeared for me. Now more absence. She'd been up for Christmas, just two weeks earlier in her dress-up red velveteen sweats. She scooted next to me on the couch and asked me to tie her red and white handkerchief around her neck.

"I can't get it right," she said, lifting her chin in that nose-in-the-air gesture she had as I fiddled with it. It was her way of having me do something for her, involving me in the intimacy of dressing her, making me the mother to her needs. She did this often, asking her daughters to be the parent, which is why her ministrations to me in the last year— sending checks and cards and love, just what I needed—meant so much.

I can't absorb the fact that Sunday the fifth had been her last day of life, the day my friends came for an after-New Year's lunch since I could-n't join them for our usual Christmas Eve dinner. Her neighbor had noticed her gardening that day. I can see her in baggy cotton pants feed-ing her Brandy roses and pulling dead blossoms from the blue bache-lor's buttons out front, or raking the brittle leaves of the California live oak shading her small backyard, their needled edges grazing her palms. I can imagine her pausing to pluck the wooly leaves of pineapple sage and rub them under her nose, releasing the fruity herb scent she loved. Her physicality doesn't evaporate so quickly. Only the day before, Saturday the fourth, I'd gotten one of her full-of-mistakes, stream-of-consciousness letters typed on the old Olympia that always sat on her dining room table, papers scattered around. Mom didn't write a letter so much as send off in rapid fire her incomplete musings, enigmatic turns of thought, with a scattershot of daily itinerary and trivia. Among the outpouring was mention of a New Year's Day visit with my ninety-five-year-old paternal grandmother, who lives in a retirement home a short distance from Mom's place. Mom jotted a hasty postscript in black pen: "I have another story to relate re. your grandmother (next time I write)."

A few days later I call my grandmother—her voice quavering but clear—to prod out of her some details of that last visit with Mom, trying to get a hint of what they might have talked about. Grandma doesn't have much to say. My mother's last message swallowed away.

Death is hazy and intangible, hard to fathom, while here in my bedroom the phone is buzzing—family, friends, commiserations, warm voices. Bill tiptoes around with special care, gives me hugs and backrubs and generous looks. He drops bundles of mail and condolence cards on my quilt. I hold in my hands more letters, the ones that arrive when my mother's stop. In these notes, the message is clear and unmistakable.

In a peculiar way, I'm less alone than I've been in a long time. Everyone had worried, I later learn, that I would regress, that grief would take my body down with it, immobilize me further. It doesn't. My bed is switchboard central. The French have a word for this, "*flaneur*," the man who conducts business in pajamas and bedroom slippers, that title—hinting at flannel and flamboyance—infusing the sedentary life with not only approbation but style.

Well, the style we can set aside. But mourning has set me among the approved, accepted, and officially titled. This is a calamity everyone understands. It's one that has prescribed rituals and ready phrases and Hallmark cards. It's not uncharted territory. The pain of a mother's death is legitimate and shared and communal. No one gawks in uncomfortable silence. No one doubts. Others tell their stories and listen to mine and that miasma of misunderstandings and jagged connections that has accompanied my illness fades away.

But not the pain. Dreams and death and illness and an undercurrent of Mom's presence meld into a jumble of days spiked by a disquiet always on the edge, raw and sharp. It's fair to say I've had enough of disappearance. Lisa, too, has slipped away, clearing out her studio a few months earlier to set up housekeeping in an apartment in San Francisco with three friends. Thankfully, her defection doesn't breed absence but a burst of vitality. Her visits home have the magnanimous energy of her new freedom, full of solicitous smiles.

We stand in the backyard, a pale sun on our faces. Lisa points to two white butterflies cavorting in tandem. They swoop and dodge in great flying arcs, cutting a loopy path through the bony, ash-gray branches of our plum tree, to damp beds of azalea to clumps of spiky daylilies.

She links her arm around my waist. "Makes me think. . . ."

I tilt my head to hers and give a squeeze. She feels it, too, this inability to look at one thing without thinking of another, feeling a second presence, a shadow life glinting around us. I've been sharing my nighttime visitations with Lisa—the ethereal not Bill's forte—and she nods as if this were in the natural order of things. Of course.

I find myself gazing at flowers each day on my walk—I'm up to three blocks. A clump of violently violet cineraria pealing its noise in the shade, or my neighbor's roses, streaked pinks, magentas, oily whites. I feel an intense need for this vibrancy and color. What is it about the blaze and spectacle—there's no other word for it, really—of a flame-orange nasturtium? Stendhal called beauty a promise of happiness. I experience it as a transport system with the instant ability to distract and reassure.

At my most ill I had stared at pictures of flowers. I had discovered on my bookshelf an old hardback my mother must have given me,

The Pocket Encyclopedia of Indoor Plants. A red sticker on the front announced the sale price of $2.98. So like her. Inside were delicately drawn, full-color portraits of hibiscus, abutilon, ficus, cymbidium, lantana. The detailed illustrations and rhythmic names gave me something to focus on besides pain. I ran my finger over the curled green leaves of prayer plant, veined with cream like a butterfly wing, or the linen-smooth lip of calla lily. Prayer plant, calla lily. I loved the names.

My mother, an avid gardener, had had at her command this rangy, lyrical vocabulary of flowers. When we strolled through the neighborhood, as she loved to do, she'd name each plant, bending to touch or pointing a finger or tipping her eye. My mother knew something not just about flowers but about a certain rhythm or pace of life that allowed for the time to pause and look and attach a name to what she saw.

My inflamed brain demanded just this quiet focus: flowers, soup, clouds. I don't think it was an accident that I was drawn to that sturdy women's gardening book when my head was packed with some grainy, dense substance. I couldn't read, couldn't think. Flowers were what I could still have. I took them in like heat or light, without effort. I let the pages fall open and gazed into this fantasy world, bugless and unsoiled, as removed from the "real" world as my own life had become, as elegant as mine was messy. "Dancing girl" begonia with its tossed arches of curled, silvery pink leaves. Blue-bell cups of trumpet vine. Morning glory. I imagined someone laboring over the line drawings, absorbed in each crenelated petal, just as I now was. That absorption in beauty was what I needed.

In those intense, early months of my illness, my sister Suzanne carried in a stem of gladiola buds, its cut tip wrapped in tinfoil. Bill set it in a nubby glass vase on my oak lowboy dresser. I watched the buds, tight as corn husks, unfurl on their stalk one by one over a course of days, into a spread of ruffled, showy pink-orange. That flowering held my attention for long stretches of time.

I know one woman who, deathly ill from cancer, wailed, "I never want to see another goddamn flower!" It's strange to think what potent symbolic force a simple object possesses in the face of illness. For me, that single bloom was something to hang onto, like a valued family vase taken into a new country, a reminder that the world left behind can in some small way be retained. Its unfolding seemed to me a note of faith, proof of something steady and in its place.

It wasn't just beauty I craved, but the order beauty implies. I longed for a sunlit room, uncluttered, a smooth quilt. A spray of roses and dusted furniture. I needed an ordered loveliness to counter the biochemical melee raging in my body, the impotence I felt in the face of my body's collapse. I wanted an ideal world, suspended and safe, all the cacophony and debris of illness swept away. As Lynne Sharon Schwartz wryly notes in her novel about a woman with chronic fatigue syndrome, "Restoring order may be the tangible expression of panic, but it's also the remedy."[1]

I've heard other people who are ill express this sentiment: the desire to clean out cupboards and closets, scrub floors in the face of illness, to control what we can—though such industry wasn't exactly a priority for Bill and Lisa, stumbling in with my chicken noodle soup and hot compresses and laundry, overworked and stressed. I found beauty where I could, in the copper light infusing the leaves of our Japanese maple, like clusters of tiny illuminated umbrellas. Illness, like grief, carries its own imperative, to seek the serenity and simplicity that can heal. "Getting well," Marc Barasch sagely notes, "may be less a matter of fighting illness, than of counter-balancing it with the healthy aspects of our lives."[2]

Several months after my mother's death, my friend Susan H. sweeps into the living room for my birthday lunch, ashimmer in gold-threaded indigo pants and bangled bracelets. There's a swirl of hugs and exclamations—"Oh, you look great"—bags and presents. Before we settle on the couch for kung pao chicken, she bends over the coffee table and pulls from her leather tote bag a book by photographer and artist Andy Goldsworthy.

"Have you seen? . . . Isn't he amazing?" Besides bringing energy, friendship, a reason to put on a skirt and blue chenille scoop-necked top, she's brought me a trip to a museum in the comfort of my living room. I can't tell her how much this means.

I pounce on the book, paging through the photos as if a window has opened. Goldsworthy's photos of natural objects—leaves, stones, ice—arranged in a natural setting as provocative sculptures captivate me: a braid of yellow leaves snaking through a shaded gully, a precariously balanced tower of stones in a rocky field, nature manipulated to show-case nature, sinuous, suggestive. What is lasting? What ephemeral? In one picture, a sliver of ice balances precariously on ice. Its striking pose lived only the instant it took to snap the camera, then survived indefi-nitely as artifice.

I'm starved for this stimulation that takes me beyond the limits of my room, my house. If beauty, like love, can calm and reassure, it can also alert and stimulate. A stream of yellow leaves, like a woven mat of water, or a single jagged edge of chalky limestone whose rough powder I can almost feel between my fingers. There is something visceral, bodi-ly, about beauty, as if jolting me on an electro-chemical level, recoordi-nating the discordant waves in my brain, aligning something that was jangled, the way pendulums set to swinging at random will gradually synchronize. Whatever it is, I feel touched.

Perhaps this response is the body's way of ensuring that illness is about more than a down-regulated hypothalamic-pituitary-adrenal axis or increased cytokine levels, that something else stays in the illness equa-tion, something ineffable and intangible and, well, soulful. Or perhaps it's the other way around, as the field of psychoneuroimmunology sug-gests: the environment, mental imagery, even a flower, create mood-induced changes in the nervous system, causing it to release neurochemicals that in turn affect the immune system, producing improved health. We are a mass of chemicals after all.

As an ill person, I'm a staunch empiricist. Whatever works is all I need to know. I leave it to the purveyors of energetics, healing vibrations, and aromatherapy, the biochemists and molecular biologists, to figure out the mechanism, which apparently they're a long way from doing. But I know this: it would be a mistake to think of beauty as luxury, the first thing to be dispensed with in times of crisis. The more ill or pained I was, the more essential it seemed.

As I've become stronger, the importance and solace of beauty never lessen. The colors of leaves—yellows, cinnabar, auburn, like teas—hold my attention every day. "Every now and then, in my waking moments, and especially when I am in the country, I stand and look hard at everything," writes William Maxwell in his essay "Nearing Ninety."[3] Illness, like age, or a death, invokes loss and a desire to absorb intensely what one still has. I, too, want to stop and stare for long moments, to keep those colors with me.

A thing of beauty is something that is not final. You can return to it again and again and still be absorbed, drawn into its details and shadows and questions. It is never finished or exhausted. It calls you back. In this sense it is the opposite of the neatness and order I craved. It provides an escape from the need for safe harbor, assuring a world not encased or limited by those needs. It holds promise of something more to come.

14

That Name.2

[The name] chronic fatigue syndrome just doesn't cut it. . . . People don't really understand how [CFS] can destroy someone's life. It's not fatigue. It's far, far worse than most people can even imagine.

—Laura Hillenbrand, quoted in *The CFIDS Chronicle*

March 1997

On a warm spring day, I defect from my HMO, leaving it to the grander tasks of surgery and CT scans, and head once again to the office of an acupuncturist, finally feeling strong enough to try someone friends have recommended. I'm greeted by a woman who is a cross between a cherub and a Buddha, with tight blond curls and a Southern accent. I have the feeling I'm in for something interesting. She squints at my throat as if trying to decipher enigmatic road signs, probes my shoulder blades, and taps needles into my earlobes. It makes as much sense to me as anything else. She seems to know the subterranean pathways this illness travels, her office walls hung with diagrams of human bodies measured by meridians and studded with pulse points. Her fingers, playing my wrist like the keys of a flute, measure pulses I can't feel. She stares blankly into space as she does this, and I imagine her envisioning my body as an illuminated *chi* flowchart—moving fine here, some congestion there, kidney, liver, lung.

The treatments only make me more exhausted, and the whole ordeal—the twenty-minute drive there and back, sunk in the passenger seat, the walk from the parking lot, down a hall, and up a flight of stairs, the talking and exertion—takes me anywhere from five days to two weeks to recover from. I continue going anyway, if only because this woman speaks a language of the body that makes sense to me. She nods knowingly at my symptoms, doesn't seem to find unusual the intractable exhaustion, the constantly abraded throat, the monotony of my complaints. My Southern Buddha doles out herbs and supplements that mute perimenopausal symptoms and allergies and help me sleep, but the underlying illness seems to heal at its own pace. I'll spend thousands of dollars on this biweekly ritual over the years. It later occurs to me this is the premium I have to pay for someone who speaks a language that takes in the whole mysterious, elusive phenomenon of the body.

The language of bioscience is another story. By 1997, the name-change movement that advocates had thought would come to a quick conclusion in the late 1980s was turning into a protracted, messy saga of patient anger and bureaucratic intransigence. On September 5, 1996, it seemed the name-change proponents had finally achieved a breakthrough. After much advocacy work and with the help of Dr. Philip Lee, Assistant Secretary for Health, a charter was signed to form the Chronic Fatigue Syndrome Coordinating Committee (CFSCC), operating within the Department of Health and Human Services, to better coordinate the response to CFS among various agencies.[1] Though the name change was not initially the focus, committee member Dr. Anthony Komaroff insisted this was a sufficiently important topic that it needed to be on every agenda. Finally, in the fall of 1998, a workgroup within the CFSCC was formed to come up with a set of criteria by which a new name could be judged. A decade after the CDC officially recognized CFS, the wheels of government were slowly grinding forward.

In April of 1999, the workgroup tackling the name-change issue developed criteria for a new name. In a bow to the inextricable entanglement of patients and the medical establishment, they acknowledged that any name change "must have the support of prominent members of the medical and research communities."[2] The criteria—which emphasized that the name should no longer focus on fatigue and that it should be evidence-based and supported by conventional scientific methods—were forwarded to then–Secretary of Health and Human Services Donna Shalala. A second workgroup within the CFSCC was charged with making a recommendation for a new name by November 2001.

Yet these painfully slow incursions into government meeting rooms did little to quell patient ire. The name-change story had become both more sedate and more volatile. As bureaucrats subdued the issue into periodic memos and surveys, the patients, for whom nothing had changed, became more obsessed than ever. Exhausted patients were still lining up at the mike at scientific meetings to demand a name change, some falling asleep in the aisle after giving their heartrending testimony of lost jobs, bankruptcy, divorce. Thomas Hennessy was still exhorting physicians and patients alike. In the spring of 2001, RESCIND and the National CFIDS Foundation circulated a petition urging the recognition of myalgic encephalomyelitis (ME). Accompanying many of the signatures were the familiar, wrenching pleas: "Please give this horrible illness a name that professionals can respect." "I've suffered for 20 years from ME. Don't insult me any further by calling it fatigue." "JUST DO IT!"[3]

Exasperated with petitions and bureaucracies, in a no-holds-barred action, an anonymous group called No Time to Lose planned an outrageous operation to be executed by May 12, 2001, the official Awareness Day for CFS. They urged those with CFS to let public officials know they intended to donate blood, saying, "If the government won't help PWCs, and science can't seem to help PWCs, then it is time for the PWC community to help itself in a way never before attempted."[4] Their plan was a deliberate attempt to contaminate the public blood supply with the blood of CFIDS patients, complete with clandestine mail drops and anonymous couriers. If public officials objected, it would be proof they knew CFS to be a serious and communicable disease. Desperation crossing into lunacy? Perhaps.

What moves and pains me as I page through the transcripts and reports that Bill pulls off the Web for me is the passionate tenacity of all these efforts and the poignancy of such extraordinary energy expended on a name. I can't get out of my mind the hundreds, perhaps thousands, of hours countless people have spent in offices and conference rooms debating a word, parsing a prefix. Or the regularly held name-change forums, at which the pleas and angst have become so depressingly familiar as to seem choreographed. One infuriated man, fed up with friends and family who think a folk remedy can fix things, demanded a name that was "popularly incomprehensible, preferably a close derivation from ominous sounding Latin roots."[5]

"Why all this noise and fuss? Why all the urgency, uproar, anguish and exertion?" mused Schopenhauer, considering love. He answered his own query. "It is no trifle that is here in question; on the contrary, the importance of the matter is perfectly in keeping with the earnestness and ardour of the effort."[6] At stake, he says, is nothing more or less than the continuation of the species. To understand the drive for love is to comprehend the fear of extinction. The fear of disappearing.

The great passions that drive the name-change movement ride on a similar, and no less biologically driven, fear. To be seen is to exist, to have presence. The great fear of the ill is erasure, to be unseen in our suffering—invisible to science, tucked away in our bedrooms. I think of all the PWCs to whom I'm now linked, electronically and bodily. The former college teacher who spends her days in one room, too exhausted to do more than maneuver between computer and daybed. Or the former health educator whose health has deteriorated for twenty years and who is now bedridden. All the PWCs in their rooms. I'd like to stretch out a map and pin a bright red flag for every sequestered, unseen person, a stark marker for all their isolation, invisibility, deprivation, for all the insults, frustration, loss. This immeasurable suffering cannot be redeemed or reversed until it is seen as Schopenhauer saw the passions of love: a matter of such importance as to be worthy of all its exhortations and furor.

You'd think the climax of this story would be the selection of a new name. Not so. In October 2001, in a moment that has to rival Y2K for anticlimax, the name-change workgroup within the CFSCC with little fanfare unveiled its recommendation for a new name: chronic neuroendocrineimmune dysfunction syndrome, or CNDS. The most common reaction was "Huh?" My own: you must be kidding.

Clumsy and lackluster as it was, it did meet the important criteria the workgroup had established. It did not imply a causative agent, since this remains unknown. It reflected the major symptoms patients report and was supported by studies in the medical literature. It also provided an umbrella term under which subgroups of patients could be identified, such as "CNDS, orthostatic intolerant–predominant"—a way to acknowledge and organize the varied patient symptoms.

Reaction was swift and mixed as ever. While 65 percent of people—mostly patients—responding to a CFIDS Association questionnaire agreed that the term CNDS was acceptable (the first word, "chronic," would later be dropped at their suggestion), the majority of researchers remained opposed to any name change.[7] And along with the questionnaires, the CFIDS Association received the much-circulated petition demanding the recognition of ME, now with 3,500 signatures. In 2002, in a we're-fed-up-with-this-prissing-around move, a group of patients announced the formation of a new advocacy group, the Myalgic Encephalomyelitis Society of America.[8] Patient divisions remained forceful and intact.

Meanwhile, the Chronic Fatigue Syndrome Advisory Committee (CFSAC) within the Department of Health and Human Services, the group slated to take up the name-change issue, stalled for nearly *three years*, during which the committee was reconfigured. Then, in an abrupt move that stunned the CFIDS community, on December 8, 2003, at their second meeting, the advisory committee flatly refused to adopt the proposed name neuroendocrineimmune dysfunction syndrome (NDS), saying, "We feel that a change of this name to another name should occur only when there is a better understanding of the pathophysiology of the illness."[9]

The CFIDS Association, noting that "the lack of scientific knowledge concerning the pathophysiology of this illness is the direct result of inadequate federal support for CFS research," urged the committee to review its position.[10] And in a disheartening admission, in 2004, the board of directors of the CFIDS Association wrote, "The CFSAC's decision means that efforts to pursue a name change stand little chance right now of succeeding beyond the patient community."[11] Meanwhile, working with the CDC, the CFIDS Association began preparing a media campaign to broaden awareness of the severity and complexity of CFS. While this may seem like a way to take direct action, in fact, changing perceptions of CFS through public education means that the name CFS will become more solidified in the public mind.

When I survey the name-change landscape today, I see a strewn battlefield, a mess. A sobering lesson in the failure of both radicalism and moderation. Working within government channels—endless meetings, endless surveys, statements, memos, position papers, haggling—produced no results. The more activist patients are still operating on the fringes and taking things into their own hands. Many are self-naming. One woman says she has RNase-L enzyme dysfunction disorder, or REDD. Others use the name postinfectious fatigue syndrome, PIFS.

Some say they have atypical multiple sclerosis. Many use ME or CFS/ME or ME/CFS. If skeptics have trouble with the idea of CFS, they're going to have a field day with this confusion.

Like many patients, I'm outraged that a name with a clear precedent in the medical literature—either epidemic neuromyasthenia or benign myalgic encephalomyelitis—or a comparably medical-sounding name, wasn't adopted at the get-go, a move that would have saved hundreds of thousands of people untold misunderstanding and dismissal over the last fifteen years. Since the publication of the Canadian clinical case definition for ME/CFS in 2003, I've become intrigued, like many, with the idea of using this dual name, which retains the name recognition of CFS and adds the gravitas of ME. Though the U.S. definitions for these two conditions differ, the existence of the Canadian definition bolsters the justification for combining the names until the mainstream scientific establishment sanctions a name change.

But what bothers me most about the name-change tug-of-war is our dependence on the medical establishment to gain recognition, credibility, and help, the power and authority biomedicine has to shape our illness experience. We shouldn't have to exhibit a biomarker or pathogen, or die, to be taken seriously. Those of us with CFIDS and other possibly overlapping chronic illnesses—Gulf War syndrome, chronic candidiasis, multiple chemical sensitivity, fibromyalgia—should be seen as what we are: emblems of the limits and weaknesses of a pathology-oriented, reductive bioscience.

The authority of scientific medicine to validate or invalidate our experience, to alienate us from what we experience in our bodies, and to give or deny a diagnosis that will bring or undermine social support constitutes too great a concentration of power. Whose interests are served when disease categories are constructed? What responsibility do doctors, researchers, and insurers have to the patient when they interpret or define that person's illness? What are the consequences of constructing diagnostic models that rely heavily on objective data and min-imally on patient experience? In what ways do technology and biologi-cal knowledge create rather than resolve problems of diagnosis? How are disease concepts and definitions influenced by the state of techno-logical development, the emergence of medical specialties, the current norms and assumptions of medical practice? These are the kinds of eth-ical questions that must be included in physician education and raised as a hallmark of twenty-first-century medicine.[12]

Medical advance is rarely an overnight event, and perhaps all the slogging through the mud, the discouragement and acrimony, will have its own slow harvest: a recognition by an increasing number of scientists and physicians that we need to acknowledge the imprecision and vagaries of medical science. We need to recognize that labs may perform only limited, standard procedures; doctors aren't always up-to-date on research; providers bring their own biases to the clinical encounter; medical training and managed care can discourage reflection, curiosity, and original thinking. We need to view illness as not only objective sci-ence but subjective experience, and to see the advances of science as tools to be used with, not instead of, clinical insight and intuition.

Yet as medical practice becomes more evidence-based, more molec-ular in focus, this convergence of nineteenth-century clinical wisdom with twenty-first-century biotechnology is less and less likely to hap-pen.[13] Even with the pressures of complementary and alternative health movements, patient advocacy efforts, and the Internet as a source of lay empowerment, the laboratory-focused biomedical model remains a powerful force to reduce patient input and authority.

I hope as fervently as anyone that the triumphal view of science will prevail, that bioscience will find the key to CFIDS and other confound-ing illnesses, discover effective treatments, and develop a cure. Yet even if biomedicine confirms an underlying disease process for CFIDS, we will still end up in the same old ill-fitting marriage between an acute-care, technological medical practice and a complex chronic illness. We will still be under the spell of a simplistic dichotomy in which diseases with a visible pathology are considered real and others are not.

Ensconced in my bedroom, I find the machinations of government committees, the turf wars and career struggles of researchers, the internecine wars of patient advocates, the foot-dragging and contention to be distant, even bizarre events. Those of us who are ill are in a strange position: we're experts on this illness, yet have no institutional authority. We appropriate scientific language—a lot of brain-fogged patients can give a dazzling spiel on RNase-L pathways and HPA axis abnormalities—but have made only minimal inroads against physician skepticism. We read up on our illness but must go for treatment to physicians who know less than we do. We struggle daily with the implications of language, but have only marginal power to affect how language is used.

The name chronic fatigue syndrome, for me, has a meaning that is profoundly personal. Its meaning is both large and sweeping—encompassing a radically altered, homebound life—and intimate and sensory, minutely focused: whether I can walk across a room without my knees wilting under me, whether I can talk on the phone for half an hour. It means I live with a constant divide between what is and what was supposed to have been.

The phone rings this April morning, 1997, three months after my mother died, with bad news. I twist over to my bedside table to grab the receiver. Solicitous, fumbling with apology (what automatic guilt illness induces in others), a kindly woman informs me that she is the new owner of my office building and I will have to move out. I'm stunned. My landlord never told me the building was for sale. The cad! He's been penuriously collecting my rent all these months, knowing I'm ill, and knowing I'll never use the office again.

I flop back on the pillow. Another loss. But I'm madder at the devious owner than at the usurpation of my office. The office, strangely, seems like an old skin I'm meant to slough off. I'm sad but not devastated. I wouldn't have given it up on my own, but it's not hard to convince myself it's for the best—I can't afford to keep paying for an office I don't use. It's curious how readily acceptance comes, as if some part of me is relieved to be unburdened, ready to pare my life to a manageable scale.

Lisa drives me over one Sunday afternoon in May to say a final good-bye. I'm not up for much, but I can't let my office disappear without a final viewing. As always, the step into the outside world catches me with pleasure. Tired as I am and despite the funereal aspect of our mission, it's invigorating to be released from enclosure, to retrace my short commute through the familiar Berkeley side streets and neighborhoods. Lisa and I don't talk much. I soak in the sunny day, the exhilarating spring air.

Shingled houses and blossoming yards. Clumps of clover draped with fallen petals of tulip trees, like paper boats. Wooden fences heavy with bursts of white jasmine. I lap up every detail with greedy attention. "Drive slow," I say. (Later I remember my mother telling me that this is what her mother said as, dying from colon cancer, she was driven to Cottage Hospital for the last time, trying to hold onto the world.)

We turn into the Shattuck Avenue business district, past Viking Trader Furniture, Good Guys electronics, emblems of my old life. Ruby's photocopy shop around the corner from my office that I used to dash into, exhausted, before meeting a client. The mailbox on the corner I had praised every day for its convenience. These two mundane fixtures in particular hold a sad resonance. They had been the shaky basis of my teetering life. The convenience of the photocopy shop and mailbox, within a block of my office, literally allowed me to manage my work life. Had they been farther away, requiring a separate errand, I don't know what I would have done.

Lisa drops me off in front of the office building—an old wooden structure that shakes when a heavy truck rumbles by, housing a suite of offices above a restaurant—then goes to park. I climb the dim, carpeted stairway to the second-story landing, wander through the hall, peer into the four other offices briefly, then open the door to my small room. At once its familiarity, its intimacy, brings a rise of joy, pride, and sadness the way a fragrance does, with an instant sweep of memory experienced in my whole body.

I thought the room would seem smaller than I remembered—isn't that the way it's supposed to be when revisiting the past?—but it seems larger, and full, though it has sat unused for twenty months. I settle in the white wicker chair in the corner, the observer now, observing my own past, taking in the nine-by-eleven, blue-carpeted room, the L-shaped desk topped by custom-made oak bookshelves (I'd bought them secondhand, though they fit my desk perfectly, one life sliding neatly into another). Stacks of thick manuscripts, computer disks, and battered folders. Packed floor-to-ceiling bookcases along one wall that my clients would stare at absently as they related their latest confusions over their stories. Several framed poems and a poster announcing a poetry reading. A small northern window overlooking an alleyway. The green swivel chair at my desk where I would lean back, gesticulating, knee to knee with my client.

I'm amazed at how much has fit into this room, all the stories that have passed through this small space. I spent ten years here, building my writing consulting business, with clients who became more than clients, fellow writers and journeyers. They'd come in clasping their pages, unfurling all the strange moments that comprise a life, surprising, painful, chilling, touching. Beyond the story on the page I'd always be witnessing a second story: The woolen-skirted schoolteacher who burst into tears when I told her her novel still needed work, and who later, after drying her eyes and corralling her rambling plot, won an NEA award. The elegant and contained fiction writer who eked out a few punishing but beautifully written pages every couple of weeks. Scanning the wall above my head one day, she told me she had pancreatic cancer—her doctor had advised her to go ahead and drink her finest wine—yet she not only lived to finish her novel, but survived the cancer. The two CIA agents in officious blue suits and dark glasses, seated stiffly—they seemed as startled by me as I did by them. What the hell, I thought, and took my pencil to their quite wooden mystery novel. Or the intense young Czechoslovakian man who read aloud an impassioned riff about the 1989 Velvet Revolution so stunningly written I could only say keep writing, and whom I never saw again.

Lisa leans in the doorway. Her sweater hugs her midriff, and I catch the glint of her belly ring. "You OK?"

"Yeah." I'm surprised at my own equanimity, at the way feelings of disruption and completion seem to merge.

The other story here is my own, of my travels from neophyte to established editor, from the time when friends came to help patch and paint what formerly had been an insurance office, when my shelves held only a few new folders, to this much-used, crammed room, thick with words. Above my desk stretches a shelf of pristine books my clients have published—novels, memoirs, nonfiction—in their glossy jackets, a stack I watched grow with the pride of a mother for her brood.

Even though I've settled into working at home, as long as I paid rent and Bill made his twice-weekly trips to pick up my mail, this office remained a vision in my head of some past still remaining, some future I would soon enter. It never occurred to me I wouldn't see clients here again. I've held fast to the vision of this room as something I still possessed, despite all evidence to the contrary, despite the fact that I speak to clients while lying in bed, the phone clasped to my ear, eyes closed, my brain straining to put together a coherent, insightful line of words, and somehow, thrillingly, managing to. At any rate, it doesn't seem to bother my clients that their angst and confusions are now spoken to the air in front of them, not much different than before.

We have a janitorial service at the office, and I'd told the service they didn't need to clean my room except for once a month or so just to keep the dust from settling. The room has been bypassed as business goes on around it, rather like the life of the ill. Anytime I wanted I could picture it as it was and know it remained intact, nothing changed; even the fingerprints of the person who broke in one night are still imprinted on the ocher metal filing cabinet where the thief filched a sheet of stamps but found nothing else of value.

A small room like this, I think, is the perfect place for nostalgia, everything contained and kept as it was. For twenty months it has sat untouched, waiting for my return. I don't really feel nostalgic; rather, I'm struck by how much this room feels like mine, and that it was mine and now isn't anymore.

"Do you want the shelves?" I had asked the new owner, who will transform my office into a reception area for her jazz school. "No, take them."

We don't stay long. I carry downstairs my electric teapot and tray of solid-colored ceramic mugs. Lisa follows with a framed photograph, given me by a client, of pastel-streaked rocks. She'll come back tomorrow to box everything up for the movers. It's not the end of my business. I'll continue working from home. But it is the end of an era, for my work and for myself.

15

On Determination

In August 1921 Franklin D. Roosevelt was stricken with infantile paralysis. By indomitable courage, iron will-power, supreme determination, he emerged triumphant—strengthened in the fires of adversity for the task ahead.

—movie newsreel in 1930s

It wasn't until my grandmother died—in 2001 at age 102—that I heard the story of the Pierce Arrow, a classic tale of triumph over adversity with just enough Yankee ingenuity to make it charming. A single parent in 1941, she wanted to go to her oldest daughter's graduation at Northwestern but didn't have the money. Nonetheless, she cleaned out her bank account, and she and her younger son and daughter climbed onto the train. They ate sandwiches they'd brought in a straw basket, slept sitting up. After the ceremony Grandma went out and bought a used Pierce Arrow with a jumpseat and glass partition, drove the family back to Santa Barbara in fine style, then promptly sold the car, earning enough to pay for the whole trip.

This story doesn't surprise me, but it's not the whole picture. My grandmother's determination was larger than that sweet tale. It had the force of a gale, powerful enough to shape her children, even her grandchildren, in that determined way mothers have: you will learn what I think important.

Hers was a determination almost vengeful in its relentlessness and always victorious, or so she thought. If ants swarmed over the sticky cin-

namon buns she was to serve me, her visiting granddaughter, for breakfast, she'd scrape and pluck them off and set in front of me on her
sparkling yellow saucer a pocked and tortured roll, as if there was no
question about it. The ants would not win in her world, not ever. Never
mind my horrified conviction that you can't tell the body parts of an ant
from a gooey streak of cinnamon.

It was Depression-era-bred frugality, of course, but it carried a whiff
of combat, an intimation of long siege—those years of divorce, single
parenthood, managing on pennies, but *managing.* I can still hear her
high, warbling voice reading to my sisters and me the chugging refrain
of *The Little Engine That Could,* that classic parable of perseverance: "I
think I can, I think I can." I remember staring at the cartoon-sketch of
the wide-eyed little train with languid, feminine lashes. Definitely
female, but with a hidden ferocious reserve. If the little engine carrying
her huge load—too big for her, you could plainly see—could make it to
the top of the hill, so could we. How could we not feel swept into this
myth of infallibility with its zealous, unswerving tune?

My father read us that story too, perched on the side of our bed. He
made a great effort of huffing and puffing through the words, "I think I
can, I think I can." As the train reached the crest and gleefully glided
downhill, he exhaled the little engine's words, "I thought I could, I
thought I could, I thought I could." How he loved that. He would give
us a great, meaningful smile, slapping his feet on the floor, as if the world
were as it should be. He'd put himself through graduate school, he never
let us forget, while working and supporting a family, and so could we.
Tenacity and determination, the undercurrents that would always carry
us where we needed to go.

It's the tinge of masochism turned into a higher calling that in retrospect makes me cringe. Now I question everything. Did I love that
book because I was supposed to, or was that long-lashed, coy ferocity a
subversive code for girls that could truly lift me up? Whatever it was, I

bought it, hook, line, and sinker. That same fierce determination to overcome any obstacle was bred in me along with the admonition to eat my spinach, and taken in the same way, through the body. Raise a child as a single parent? No problem (it runs in the family, three generations). Put myself through graduate school, build a career, with no money, while ill? I can do it. "Where there's a will there's a way," my mother crooned.

In his story "The Washwoman," Isaac Bashevis Singer regards the extremes of the Protestant work ethic with shrewd, anthropological detachment. Jewish women would never do what the old, worn washwoman does, he says. She came regularly to the Jewish household to collect their linens, walking an hour and a half back home. Her fingers were gnarled, her shoulders bent and narrow. "But there was in her a certain pride and a love of labor with which the Gentiles have been blessed. The old woman did not want to become a burden, and thus she bore her burden."[1] She arrives one harsh winter day, shaking with cold. As she staggers out into the bitter freeze under her huge bundle, the young Jewish son watches her from a distance with a mix of horror and respect for her inordinate burden.

Illness brings the perspective of distance, too, distance from one's own life, an often disconcerting view. Here I am limp as a smacked fish, congealed in a sticky lethargy no amount of will can dissolve. I'm flared-up badly this November afternoon of 1997. Propped against pillows, I feel weighted with heaviness, the air a dense, gritty substance, pressing on the top of my head, my forehead, cheekbones. My skull is packed with sludge. These flare-ups, like some massive assault, usually lasting two months, hit me over and over, as if my immune system continually revs up to fight some enormous battle.

Though the dramatic tirades of my body continue, underneath it all is a slow return of strength. After two years of recovery, I have left behind those horrible days of barely being able to walk across a room. Each morning brings a brief euphoric moment, promising five to six hours of a minimally functioning brain and body. This morning, despite that all-over sick feeling, after my morning routine—a three-hour ordeal of pouring food and liquid into me, showering, and resting until I can function—I was able to spend two hours jotting coherent notes in the margins of a client's novel while sitting in my bedside chair, get my own lunch, and do a load of dishes. Small victories. By one o'clock I'm spent, in bed, relinquishing productivity and effort the way prisoners give up their belts and keys.

The late afternoon and early evening hours are the hardest, when the sun arcs west and leaves the bedroom scattered with shadow. I'm too fatigued to read. The radio is a rattle of noise, fast and confusing, TV an overwhelming jumble of commotion. I talk to Bill, or on the phone, weak, whispery conversations since my sore throat still settles in for long weeks at a time. Or I stare at the track lighting above me, strung with cobwebs, or at the Joel Meyerowitz photo that hangs on our bedroom wall of the Hartwig house on Cape Cod, empty but suffused with light, an open door leading somewhere bright.

This evening Bill is off at a seminar. Something about democratization and Third World this or that. If we're the First World, and developing countries are the Third World, what's the Second World? I asked him this once.

"The Soviet bloc."

Funny I never knew that. The great, wintry, little-known in-between. The hybrid space that disappears in conversations. I know about that place.

At least the Soviet countries were on the map. Chronic illness? It's not only squeezed out of conversations, it's unrepresented in our collective mind. Try to locate it. You can't unless you've been there. There's no public concept of this place. Not one that bears any resemblance to this universe in a room, with its dim lights and pain, heating pad and muddy herbs caked in the bottom of a shot glass.

With Bill gone I'm bored, and despite my mushy brain, can't stop myself from flipping through TV channels for diversion. Among the too-bright flashes and jangly colors, wouldn't you know, a program about disabled people leaps into focus—men and women who through their determination have forged meaningful, productive lives. A woman musician, graceful, electric, who, though deaf, performs brilliantly for large audiences; a blind lawyer who with the use of her seeing-eye dog and technology continues a successful practice; a paraplegic journalist who travels to foreign countries, even through rugged terrain, in search of his story—neat segments that transform the wreckage of disability into triumph.

I feel slapped, cheeks flaming. This show hits me hard, setting off a wave of angry sobs that has me grabbing for the tissues. It's that journalist muscling his wheelchair over a rocky hillside to get his interview, propelled by bravado and pluck, that gets me where it hurts. (It's an astonishing image when you think of it: the crippled and maimed held up as icons of American invincibility.) I'm already dazed by the cold reality that I can't muscle my way to a fuller life, and here is this show taunting me with the message that I can, I should, if I had any gumption at all. The ire of the newly converted floods through me. As if there's no such thing as determination that is foolhardy, determination that is self-defeating. As if "I can do it" is always a healthy, positive response to adversity. I think of Singer's arthritic, pale washwoman who ultimately dies under the weight of her load, that towering bundle of dirty laundry on her back, larger than she. After delivering her last load, so ill she's become ghostly, she disappears. She's not seen again.

Weak as I am, I'm furious enough to scuttle around the bedroom to find some paper and scribble a letter of protest to the producer of that TV show, full of phrases like "simplistic, triumphalist coronation of our cultural myth of can-do optimism and rugged individualism," "clichés, casting the disabled as moral lessons, windows on human nature, for good or ill," "poster-child images as unrepresentative of and oppressive to the disabled as glossy, unblemished models are to women," etc. It's unimaginative, this portrait of disability, weak on detail, lacking in squalor and confusion and terror, a cleaned-up, evangelical account.

It's as scrubbed and chiseled as all our frontier stories, Horatio Alger rags-to-riches stories, individual hero stories. As if no undergirding communal effort ever sustained these people. I pen a few more irate lines about the show ignoring the special support network, education, money, class status, or even luck that makes possible these acts of individual accomplishment. And about the way the myth of individual grit and courage obscures the need for public policy that provides adequate support services for the disabled.

Besides the show's painful reminder that all the will in the world isn't going to get me back to the office—not this year, probably not next—what angers me more deeply is my own desire for collusion with these images. I would love to be steadfast and noble, a model of disability, to ignore illness's messiness, exposures, fears. I want that heroic, stubborn narrative to be real, my own. Instead, I've been forced to see that the collapse into illness doesn't create these stories, it implodes them. I hit my nadir in those months when I was most ill and weak, when I woke one evening to find Bill gone. Panicked, I wrestled myself up from bed and struggled to the bedroom doorway before he appeared—he'd been taking out the garbage. In my underwear and torn T-shirt I grabbed him with the anxiety of an abandoned child. "I didn't know where you were!" We were both startled and confused. Who had I become? Who was this person, vulnerable, undignified? This TV segment cut to the quick of my own fears: I am not they, the heroic disabled, "supercrips" as they're called—none of us is.

A visiting friend once said, "Why can't you just try to walk a little farther each day? One block this week, two blocks next?" Her face swam in
front of me, gay and encouraging.

How could I tell her? I'm in a different country. My language, this
new language of the disordered body, makes no sense to her. It makes no
sense to me either. My original language, the one of effort and ingenuity and tenacity, the one I'm so good at, that rolls off my tongue so readily, can't be used here.

Pizza and tart apples were stacked in colorful piles on the coffee
table. I was trying to be ordinary, to have friends stop by. But I felt
wrung through with the cold and loneliness of this unseen country I live
in.

"It doesn't work that way." I struggled for words. "I'm like a car with
one piston. If you try to drive twenty miles one week, thirty the next,
you'll just blow the piston. To drive farther you need to repair the car."

I'm outside of familiar territory, in the margins. There's no cultural
representation for an enervating chronic illness like CFIDS. No valiant
image, no stouthearted icon. You'd think, with the rising numbers of
chronically ill, our cultural imagination would have expanded beyond
the heartwarming and trite. It's not just the narrowness of those TV
images—people with emphysema, heart disease, or lupus surely aren't
included. What's disturbing is the elevation of accomplishment, its dis-
tillation into the moral equivalent of valor.

We want illness to be Aristotelian: conflict, heroic struggle, resolu-
tion. A steady rise toward a victorious climax. An intrepid journalist.
Rugged terrain. Successful story. Sociologist Arthur Frank calls this culturally preferred illness story, braced by optimism and denial, the "restitution plot."[2] In this story, illness is followed by a return to health, or at
least a praiseworthy defeat of limits. These Dauntless Hero stories may
be reassuring to those who are healthy. To the ill they're an uncomfort-

able reminder that illness is a meritocracy, with virtues (accomplishment, boldness, odds-winning) and sins (silence, invisibility, a disquieting range of emotions, failing to improve).

I get tired thinking about it. I deposit the semicoherent scribbled notes to that TV producer on my bedside table and burrow back into bed.

Those of us who are ill find satisfaction where we can, in feeble protests and minor vindications. It was with no small glee that I later learned John Hockenberry, the intrepid paraplegic journalist profiled in that TV show, had had a rough time on his brazen trip through the rocky, refugee-flooded hills of Afghanistan to interview rebel fighters. In retrospect he saw it as a rather reckless adventure. It had been an enormous physical challenge, to change his catheter in a completely unsterile environment, to rely on erratic guides to carry him over steep terrain. At one point he'd been left sitting for hours, helpless, among the starving refugees, with no food or water, his blood sugar dangerously low. This is the part you don't see in these stories. The catheters. The fear. Guides who don't show up.

Illness is a lot about wandering, and about being lost. It's a venture into terrain that is sometimes wretched, ugly, disconcerting. Unfamiliar terrain, where the "I can do it" lessons of my childhood no longer take me where I need to go. The "return of the repressed," Freud called it— the reactivation of those forces, in ways we don't anticipate or control, that have been shoved underground: frailty, vulnerability, loss of control. Freud's phrase always makes me think of a grade B movie, ghoulish spirits sidling from clammy basements. And I'm the one unable to run away, rooted in a slimy muck.

My Jewish/Buddhist friend brings meditation tapes, gift-wrapped in glittery red foil. "All that time to meditate," she says with a gleam of envy, which strikes me as decidedly un-Buddhist. I give her a dark look.

It is what I do here though, in my own way, staring out my bedroom window at the fiery magenta leaves of our Japanese maple, backlit and glossy as lipstick. I never tire of this view.

"Yield," says the Tai Chi teacher to his student in Lynne Sharon Schwartz's novel *The Fatigue Artist*. The narrator, a woman with CFIDS, is watching a martial arts lesson in the park, an exercise called "push hands," in which one opponent tries to topple or dislodge another. The teacher says, "Stop relying on strength. Just try to adhere and stay balanced. You will fail many times. It doesn't matter. You are making an investment. You're investing in loss."[3]

Yield. This is my lesson, too. Stop relying on strength in order to gain strength. It feels strange to me, foreign, to bend to an opposing force rather than pushing against it. This is a different kind of determination, one that lets the opposing force pass through and by, leaving you intact rather than shattered, able to gather strength rather than dissipate it. This kind of determination can feel invisible and insubstantial, not as trustworthy or evident as that push-ahead, active, muscled determination. Our culture hasn't taught us about this second kind, has treated it as even less than a poor step-cousin, as something that doesn't exist. Our positive-thinking gurus allow no room for that tentative voice, "But maybe I need to accept. . . ." In chronic illness, the "myth of a cure," writes psychiatrist Arthur Kleinman, must be replaced by a "pragmatic notion of illness maintenance and disability reduction."[4] Rather than being a sign of giving in or defeatism, he says, this shift in attitude can increase feelings of mastery and contribute to an increased sense of well-being that in turn helps healing.

How hard it is to grapple with acceptance, a positive acceptance that will allow wise choices and an integrated sense of self, of who I am now. In *The Wounded Storyteller*, Arthur Frank points out that accepting the need for a new identity in the face of chronic illness is a way to reclaim the illness story from the restitution myth, the cheerful insistence that illness will be temporary, followed by a quick return to a productive life. The acceptance of, or at least acquiescence to, a limited life is not only a necessary adaptation, but a profound statement about illness: that it doesn't always resolve; that it can require a permanent adjustment to a less active life; that modern medicine can't always provide cures. Seen in this context, the sequestered body is rewriting the story of illness and insisting on its truth, that retreat is a gesture toward fuller health, and that in chronic illness, a full rejoining of society may not be possible.

I've struggled to shake myself awake from romanticism—the job of illness and of aging—from the rosy belief in my own endurance, the belief that I can keep going despite my body's aches and fatigue. That romanticism has a painful underside, a subtle erosion of the body's strength, like acid eating at metal, until the firm, strong support crumbles with a simple touch of the finger. "Sick people often speak of having to unlearn the habits of their upbringing in order to live well with their illnesses and heal, if possible," writes Kat Duff, who knows well the upheavals of CFIDS.[5]

Several weeks after I'd watched that TV show about the iron-willed disabled, my father sent a Christmas letter, typed on his computer, as always, in faint dot-matrix print and neatly folded in quarters. The note was two paragraphs, long for him. He is not a man of words. He wished me a Merry Christmas, encouraged me to "hang in there," and reminded me of the story of *The Little Engine That Could.* I shook my head, flooded with a tender sadness, for that distant memory of our nighttime reading, sitting shoulder to shoulder on my bed. For my father's incorrigible belief in determined possibility. For the lost world in which that belief had been enough. The glorified sentiments in that story now make me wince, like I. B. Singer's narrator watching the old washwoman sag under her burden—a measure of the distance I've traveled here in bed.

I tossed and turned that night. My hip and shoulder bones sent out shooting pains if I lay on my side. My aching toes couldn't bear the weight of the blankets if I lay on my back. My sinuses were too tender to lie on my stomach. Images of those jaunty, defiant disabled men and women played through my mind.

Other images, too, spun in their nighttime vortex: my child body leaping and flying across lawns and fences with a boundless energy and enthusiasm that now seems as distant as that childhood time. What happens to that old self, that exhilarated aliveness set aside by illness? Where is it lodged? What happens to that spirit? To body memory?

Here's another story: When I was eight, on a rare trip that I later realized was part of an unsuccessful effort to shore up their faltering marriage, my father and mother packed our blue '57 Chevy station wagon, and my older sister and I clambered in among pillows and suitcases. We set out from L.A. for a cabin at Lake Tahoe, up Highway 99 through the sweltering Central Valley, into the red-earthed, winding mountain roads. It was a happy time before the rupture to come. One hot day we set out on a nine-mile hike, forging our way over a rocky trail through magnificent bluish-green sugar pine and huge granite boulders that looked blasted from an apocalyptic explosion, down through moist gullies and snaking tree roots, steeped in dusty forest smells. I had never been so lost in a place, in the good sense of lost, in which things as you know them are replaced by a wild, spacious landscape wondrously new and appealing.

Down a ravine we stopped for a rest amid a circle of stately ponderosa pines, one of those magical spaces shaped by the death of a tree, when the ring of opportunistic roots sends up shoots. The air was refrigerator cool on my face. I found a granite rock with an upright slab behind it, a ready-made chair, and laid my cheek against the cold stone. I fit the forest perfectly. At that moment the woods seemed made for wandering and rest, for quiet immersion in the brittle scent of pine nee-

dles, the coiled vines, spurs of bark, and dense, vegetative decay. I wanted to sit and dream for hours, my cheek against that rough granite, staring into the distant light-hazed patterns of sky and branch.

After ten minutes, my father with military precision was up and
ready to go. He is not a particularly athletic man. A mathematician, he
is tall and thin with the long fingers of an artist. But when focused on a
task, he is unerringly purposeful. I was still tired. To my protests he
responded cheerily, "You can stay if you want." He, my mother, and sister took off down the trail. I knew he meant it. They weren't going to
wait. We'd rested long enough. I dragged myself up.

An hour or so later he gave a pleased, head-wagging chuckle as I
raced ahead of him in my plaid pedal-pushers shouting, "I got a second
wind," as indeed I had. What delight he felt at this confirmation: we all
have great capacity that we will discover only by pushing ourselves.

Here in the uncomfortable hold of illness, I again have the freedom
to sink into an imaginative drift. My illness-forced immobility is hardly
a forest-drunk immersion in a found world, but the thought is there: my
interruption from determined, plow-ahead activity has returned me to
that airy landscape of treetops and sky, released me to the exploration
that happens when you're not called away, when you're left to meander.

I still feel a restless chafing and frustration, an inner struggle, a kind
of "push hands" within myself as my spirit and desire strain against the
reins of my body. Determination checked by fatigue, spirit checked by
body, body urged on by spirit, that exuberant child. I'm still wandering
in this place called illness, trying to find my way, through a strange
amalgam of surrender and striving, that curious mix of new lessons and
old we're always trying to calibrate as we step forward. I like that Tai Chi
teacher's phrase: investing in loss. I suppose that's what we do all our
lives.

16

Candida Connection

By analyzing each incidence of illness as a separate occurrence, whose etiology exists only in individual minds and bodies, patterns of circumstance, especially environmental causes such as pollution or low-level radiation, have been obscured.

—Susan Griffin, *What Her Body Thought*

April 1998

I'm startled when Lisa pulls up unexpectedly one day in her battered Toyota. Just wandering back from my afternoon walk, I watch her in confusion. Why is she stopping by? Her face comes at me from across the street, shoulders hunched. Black tank top and tight jeans. She's too thin, I think.

She blurts the words mid-stride. "I have candida. I can't believe it. Candida."

"Candida?" I scrutinize the tiny lines crinkling her forehead.

Her eyes simmer with indignation. "I can't eat anything. I can't believe it. I can't eat ice cream and I can't have bread and cheese or sugar. What am I going to do? This sucks."

Then I remember. She's just been to see my acupuncturist because of her constant colds. A dawning realization, like something in peripheral vision, makes its way into focus. Of course my daughter is ill—all those colds, her low energy. Something had to have been wrong. In an instant my never fully articulated but always lurking fears come to fruition: my daughter has my bad genes or bad luck or bad karma and will be eating her wheat germ, examining her throat for white patches, and bemoaning hopeless physicians just like I do. And guilt, guilt, guilt. How could I not have known?

"Are you hungry? Here, I'll fix you lunch." I squeeze her shoulders—too small, too knobby—and lead her inside.

She slumps at the table while I whisk out hamburger, spinach, sweet potato, in full-swing mother mode, scrambling to place on her plate anything that might promise a reversal of fortune. "There's plenty you can eat, you'll see. I'll get you a candida cookbook."

"No more beer, wine. There goes my social life. What am I supposed to do when I go out with my friends? Drink water?"

Lots of things are clicking into place: not just her colds throughout college, her fatigue, but the irritability, mood swings, the light-headed, spacey feelings. No wonder.

Molds and yeasts give us wonderful things—antibiotics, beer, leavened bread, tasty mushroom-smothered steaks. These fungi can also do really bad things to plants and to the human body. Think of the 1845 Irish potato blight, caused by *Phytophthora infestans*, an organism that turned firm white potatoes to black, necrotic husks, infested shells that crumbled to the touch.

In people, candida can be an insidious guest, growing unnoticed, wreaking silent havoc. Give it a foothold and watch out. College, I now see, was Lisa's Waterloo: tossing off a latte and apricot Danish before she pulled on leg warmers and headed to the studio for morning pirouettes and leaps and bends. Before performances, a backstage candy bar pick-me-up. Keg parties on weekends. The yeast in beer, the sugary sweets, those indulgences, are what fuel candida's expansion.

When I visited the student apartment at U.C. Santa Barbara that she shared with three others her senior year in 1994, two things imprinted on my mind, besides the after-a-cyclone decor: the line of thick beer glasses on the kitchen counter and the blatantly sexual—something to do with cigars—poster in the living room. I don't remember talking about fatigue. Now she tells me how she often dragged around, sometimes barely able to get through a rehearsal. One instrumental medley with Scottish bagpipes and a techno beat kept her fast-stepping for five minutes. "I was dying," she says. "I didn't think I could do it." But she did—we cheered from the auditorium—and that effort, that shining onstage moment, that performance, kept us all blind to her body's trouble.

Candidiasis develops when a form of yeast in the bowel, *candida albicans,* normally beneficial, shifts into hyperproduction, a kind of mania on a yeasty level.[1] More than an overgrowth, it's a transformation, a shift in essence from benign to dangerous. In its proliferation, candida evolves from the yeastlike form that looks like a microscopic fried egg to the mycelial fungal form, producing rhizoids, or long rootlike tentacles, that penetrate the mucosal wall of the intestine and allow substances from the gut to leak into the bloodstream. Toxins produced by the candida, and the candida itself, run amok, gaining transport to all parts of the body and causing the symptoms of candidiasis: brain fog, joint pain, fatigue, sore throat, insomnia, irritability, bloating, indigestion. Transformed, candida becomes a threat, its expansion literally poisonous. A person can die from systemic yeast.

Most physicians regard *candida albicans* as a normal part of the body's internal flora that causes a problem only if the immune system is impaired, as in AIDS patients.[2] Physicians readily diagnose a massive yeast overgrowth and treat it appropriately with antifungal medications. Yet many alternative practitioners and some in the biomedical community believe candida can grow in the intestine and other places in the body in amounts not sufficient for diagnosis by standard Western medical practices, but enough to overburden the immune system. These subclinical problems with candida are highly controversial; many physicians believe they're overdiagnosed or nonexistent.

Like CFIDS, low-level candidiasis exists in that murky borderland of disputed and disparaged conditions. Lisa will soon be initiated into the frustrating encounter with allopathic doctors who either dismiss her candida ("It's a complete myth") or at best are open-minded but uninformed ("I really don't know that much about it, but I'd be happy to prescribe an antiyeast medication if you want me to").

Dr. Carol Jessop, who treated hundreds of Bay Area patients with CFIDS in the 1980s and early '90s, acknowledges, "It's a real no-no in Western medicine. They feel like there's no real medical proof."[3] But, she says, as more and more CFIDS patients poured into her clinic, she decided to "think outside the box" and see how they responded to antifungal treatment.[4] In fact, when she prescribed the antifungal ketoconazole and encouraged patients to clean up their diet, many improved. "I was impressed that there was a difference, and so were they."[5]

We don't know how many people have candida. We do know that many people with CFIDS and overlapping conditions such as fibromyalgia, multiple chemical sensitivity (MCS), and Gulf War syndrome also have symptoms of candida, and benefit from antifungal medications and an "antiyeast" diet: elimination of alcohol, sugar, and refined carbohydrates.[6] If we add up all the people with CFIDS and overlapping conditions who improve with such treatment, we're looking at a significant population; it likely includes millions.[7] The reluctance of mainstream medicine to take a look at this possibly widespread problem is disturbing, and telling.

To recognize and acknowledge the existence of candida in a broad population of people, not just cancer or AIDS patients, is not only a matter of acknowledging suffering and being better able to help patients. It constitutes a direct challenge to the standard biomedical account of what produces yeast overgrowth. It offers an alternative story of immune system breakdown, suggesting the immune system may be unduly taxed not just by conditions medical science recognizes—AIDS, immunosuppressant drugs—but by conditions it doesn't typically examine, such as environmental pollution or diet. This illness story proposes that aspects of our daily life thought to be innocuous—the homes we live in, the food we eat—may in fact be toxic. And if this new story of immune dysfunction is given credibility, we must look squarely at the growing problem and search for a cause. This is where acknowledging candida becomes a revolutionary act. And a complicated one, putting us back at the beginning, debating those controversial origin stories.

We know candida is often linked to a high-sugar diet, to stress, to use of birth control pills, or to overuse of antibiotics or cortisone medications. But is it also linked to our industrialized, polluted environment? The microecology of the gut can seem an uncanny reflection of the outside world. Candida, for example, produces internal mycotoxins (fungal poisons), one of which, acetaldehyde, is similar to formaldehyde and poisons the nervous and immune systems. Formaldehyde and other aldehydes are some of the most common toxins in daily life, found in everything from cosmetics to paper, particle board, plywood, and preservatives, and are a big trigger for those with multiple chemical sensitivity.

Are candida, CFIDS, and other immune system disorders—the last twenty years have seen a startling rise in lupus, MS, allergies, asthma— an early warning sign, as many believe, a sign of the vulnerability and fragility of a planet under ecological assault? Are these illnesses connected to the roughly 80,000 to 100,000 chemicals that have been poured into our environment since World War II—organophosphate pesticides, dioxins, DDT, benzene, lead, arsenic, cadmium, PCBs? Approximately 20 new chemicals are put into use each week, yet we know little or nothing about their potential health effects. Although a handful of the most dangerous chemicals have been largely eliminated from use in advanced countries—DDT, PCBs, the pesticide DBCP— even in the United States only about 15,000 have ever been tested for even one potential health effect. Among these 15,000, only 200 or so are sufficiently well characterized to determine the potential risk from exposure.[8] And even those chemicals that *are* tested are studied primarily for acute, short-term effects rather than long-term immunotoxic damage or interactions with other dangerous compounds.

A few weeks after Lisa's diagnosis, she joins me and a couple of my friends on the back deck for my birthday lunch. It's a sunny spring day. The yard is thick with a burst of leaves and buds, clumps of crimson azalea, purple crocus, honey-orange nasturtiums. The red-leafed maple arches above us, casting us in a bronze-tinged shade. These friends and I go way back. In the late 1970s, when we were young and indestructible, we stomped and rocked to Bob Marley and "Saturday Night Fever." Though the beginnings of these immunologic epidemics were in place, we were blissfully ignorant, caught up in love affairs, patchouli candles, and late night debates about the social origins of gender. Now we count around the group, not sure whether to be unnerved or dismayed, saddened or shocked. Susan, who has had asthma since childhood, battles chronic sinus infections. Rachael lives with the pain and fatigue of fibromyalgia, Lisa has candidiasis, I have chronic fatigue syndrome.

We've convened in a circle of plastic chairs on my back deck not because it's a lovely day; we have no other choice. I'm too fatigued to go to a restaurant, and Susan risks infection if she sets foot in my cat-dandered house. Our birthday ritual has become a truncated, almost comic affair. We duck into the kitchen only to fill our plates. Rachael peels the crust off her pizza because of her no-carbohydrate diet that helps her aches and pains. Lisa's diet means she can eat only vegetable soup and salad. I'm swirling with exhaustion, trying to rouse the energy for conversation, but really what I'm feeling is things slipping away. What have we come to? When my mother was my age she would not have heard of most of these illnesses, could not have had such a gathering. And we're not an aberration. Statistics reveal that an autoimmune disease affects one in five Americans and is the fourth-leading cause of disability for women.[9]

I don't know if chemicals and pollutants are behind our distress, but there's no question these toxins have worked their way into our lives, our bodies, in the name of progress and scientific advancement. I can still recall the smell of malathion—rancid and sweet, like perfume with a moldy underlayer. Summer afternoons in the 1950s, my mother, in short shorts and halter top, screwed onto the end of the hose a grimy quart-sized plastic bottle filled with dark green fluid and, as if waving a wand, wafted a filmy cloud over her camellias, Montezuma roses, and gardenias with no more thought than if she were clipping a spray of mums for the dinner table. We kids raced barefoot across the lawn, under the brackish plume filling our lungs, coating our skin. That acrid smell masked by sweetness was entwined with the frenetic, happy play of summer. We feared the atomic bomb, the Russians, dangers distant and amorphous, not the vaporous droplets falling in our own front yard.

The EPA in 2000 was about to label malathion a "likely" human carcinogen when, under pressure from the manufacturer, it backed off.[10] The engines of industry are not easily slowed. There is a self-perpetuating dynamism in complex systems, an inexorable playing out of forces already in motion. Once introduced, industrial processes and chemicals are not easily removed from use. The federal regulatory agencies—EPA, FDA—are feeble gatekeepers for an onslaught of chemicals with entrenched industrial and commercial utility.

Though many experts as well as laypersons link environmental hazards, including pesticides and industrial chemicals, to rising rates of cancer and immune illnesses, a cause-and-effect relationship is hard to establish. Roughly 80 percent of the commodities produced in this country are the result of some kind of industrial chemical process.[11] Yet we have no idea how all this commercial and chemical activity might impact our bodies. The data simply isn't there. We have data on death rates from cancer, but not on who gets cancer or what their environmental exposures have been.[12] And we have far more data on cancer than on other chronic diseases because of cancer registries that track incidence by location.

In 1999 and 2000, the Centers for Disease Control undertook the first nationwide study to measure pollution in our bodies, testing for 116 substances. The results, released in February of 2003, showed surprisingly widespread contamination with pesticides, mercury, phthalates—chemicals linked to cancer, sterility, and birth defects, and known to affect reproduction and brain development.[13] Released at the same time were the shocking results from another study, sponsored by Mt. Sinai School of Medicine in New York in conjunction with the Environmental Working Group and Commonweal.[14] In a move said to "put a human face" on the issue of environmental contamination—and underscoring a distrust of governmental agencies—a group of nine people underwent their own battery of tests. These nine people, including Michael Lerner, founder of Commonweal, had no unusual exposures to contaminants, yet each had an average of 91 pollutants in his or her body, 53 of which are linked to cancer or health problems affecting the nervous, endocrine, and reproductive systems. Michael Lerner was stunned. "Being tested yourself brings the body burden home in a very personal way."[15] He's lived for years with hand tremors, and now wonders if they might be related to some of the contaminants in his body, including mercury and arsenic.

Coming fifty years too late, these studies confirm that the body is not a closed system but intimately linked to its environment. Pollution is personal. Chemicals don't recognize borders. Carried on the wind, pesticides used in the tropics turn up in the Arctic. The dioxin spewing from a waste incinerator in Ames, Iowa, migrates on northbound weather patterns and settles into the local ecosystem of Canada's Nunavut Territory, where the Inuit eat whale and seal blubber loaded with dioxin. Traces of prescription drugs are in our rivers; pesticides are in our blood. And no one is untouched.

Fired up by the findings, in March of 2003 Lerner and several colleagues founded CHE, the Collaborative on Health and the Environment, an umbrella organization chaired by Dr. Phil Lee that now includes over 150 groups such as the California Academy of Family Physicians, the Institute for Children's Environmental Health, and the Breast Cancer Fund.[16] Bringing together health practitioners, scientists, patients, and community leaders, CHE is launching discussions about the current state of science on health and the environment. They're advocating biomonitoring to measure levels of contaminants in our bodies, and health tracking to correlate exposures and disease. Their actions underscore the shameful fact that it takes a grassroots effort of concerned citizens to push for the development of this crucial data.

"Do I have chronic fatigue syndrome?" Lisa calls from the restaurant in San Francisco where she bartends. Her voice comes in punctuated staccato over shrill laughs and bass rumbles.

I pull in a tight breath. "No," sharply, then more calm. "No. You have candida."

I'd always harbored a secret fear that somehow, through germs or genes, I might pass CFIDS on to Lisa. I would watch her lithe, mobile body, wiping hands on a towel I just used, flopping on my bed to unravel the emotional intrigues of adolescence, and wonder whether we were courting trouble, whether the innocuous exchanges of mother and daughter could be breeding ground for future disaster.

I don't tell her this. There are other things I don't tell her. That I have no guarantees. That I don't know what genetic susceptibilities wind through her DNA, what unreckoned events, what environmental stresses or bugs might worm their way into her future.

"Take your vitamins. Don't do too much." Lame clichés all I can offer, a sad, ascetic hedge against uncertainty. "What makes you ask?"

"I was reading some stuff. They're so similar." We've taken to comparing symptoms: how hormonal changes increase our brain fog and irritability. How too much talking thickens the lymph nodes and makes the lining of our throats painful and fatigued—Lisa clutches her throat to describe it and sticks out her tongue, aghhh. How our symptoms worsen if we do too much.

I remind her, and myself, of the differences, too. She doesn't have normal stamina, catches too many colds, is sometimes brain-fogged and needs extra sleep, but she leads an active life. As long as she stays on her diet and gets enough rest, she can work full-time, travel, go out with friends.

"Just take good care of yourself. You'll be OK." I feel like some CEO practicing deniability, only I don't make money as a result.

A pause, tiny exhale. "So I went out with this guy."

I hear her munching as she talks, eating dinner before her shift. Chicken with no sauce, salad with no dressing, specially made for her by the restaurant's Guatemalan cook.

"He wanted to go to a bar. I say, 'I can't drink for a while, sorry.'

"He says, 'You want to go to a restaurant?'

" 'It's really hard for me to eat restaurant food. I'm on this really strict diet right now.'

" 'Let's go to a cafe.'

" 'I can't have tea or coffee.'

"I wanted to go to a movie. He didn't want to go to a movie. And we're like, 'Ooo-Kaay.' "

"Are you feeling any better?" I ask.

"Yeah, but my social life sucks. And I'm dying for a chocolate brownie. I'm losing weight. I'm wasting away."

I read a book about a woman with undiagnosed candida who shrank to eighty pounds and became too weak to get out of bed. Her skin turned pale as wax. Strings of yellow fungus hung from the back of her throat before a doctor understood her condition. I shudder at the thought of where Lisa was headed before she was diagnosed, at the thought of all our hidden calamities.

Another thought surfaces: that we've turned on its head the traditional Chinese view of illness as payback for ancestral displeasure, punishment for the failure of the current generation to properly discharge its duties to those who nurtured them, a trope replayed every time a parent backhands an insufficiently appreciative child: "I feed you! I clothe you!" In a fateful twist, we, the soon-to-be ancestors, and our ancestors before us, are the ones not carrying out our duty to our progeny, handing them a legacy of environmental degradation and insidious sickness. Genes? Unhealthy lifestyles? Chemicals? Viruses? All of the above? I wonder what Lisa has inherited, what we're all passing along.

In 1970, when I first married, my husband and I owned a color TV, a stereo system—turntable, amplifier, two speakers—and a clock radio. Today my partner and I have two color TVs, three VCRs, one clock radio, one clock radio/CD player, two computers, two laser printers, one copier, two fax machines, three answering machines, one microwave, two stereos, two tape decks, one CD player. We've held out on a cell phone.

As a culture, we are drowning in excess, in overproduction: fertilizers, pesticides, hormones, antibiotics, industrial chemicals, plastics. We shower our systems with pharmaceuticals whose immunotoxic properties remain unstudied. We overuse corticosteroids and antibiotics, encouraging the overgrowth of yeast as well as more virulent, drug-resistant bugs. The number of vaccines we give our kids has soared, with unknown consequences. We consume too much, produce too much, accumulate too much, eat too much.

It's hard not to feel that an illness like candida is enmeshed with our cultural effusions. Isn't Lisa's candida an illness of excess, a kind of toxic spill within her body, a poisonous ebullience multiplying and spreading, leaking through boundaries, inhabiting places it shouldn't? The frightful image of candida's superabundance, its perilous profusion, is what seems to me most revealing. The gargantuan abundance of the internal flora invades and pollutes other parts of the body. It is an expansion that mirrors the unsustainable productive overkill of our culture.

I think of the weight of our acquisitions when I make out my sober shopping list: organic greens, soy milk, carrots. I wonder at the connection between my sparse, vigilantly controlled diet and this superabundance. I think of these things when I have my fatigue dreams—recurring dreams of lying prone, exhausted, while everyone is busy around me, in a theater, an office—and wake thick-headed and achy. I think of the deluge of modern life in the afternoon when I lie down to rest and my house feels full of things I haven't the energy to dust or scrub or reprogram. We have all been shaped by our excesses, our lives rearranged.

Our unquenchable appetites, voracious consumption, constantly expanding GNP, the teeming profusion of our expanding populations (projected to be over nine billion by 2050)—these are ominous extravagances. The more people, the more economic activity, the more pollution, the more chemicals lodged in our bodies. The reshaping of our inner landscape—our autonomic, neuroendocrine, and immune systems—though less visible than our cell phones and Palm pilots, may be the most profound rearrangement of our lives.

Writer Richard Preston has called AIDS the "revenge of the rainforest." We destroy the forest for its land and goods. It destroys us with its store of viruses that jump at the opportunity for a new ecological niche: our bodies. Who's to say that the rise in cancer rates and neuroendocrine and immune illnesses over the last twenty years isn't a similar revenge? The revenge of dioxin-laced waterways, contaminated lands, ozone-depleted skies. The price of our appetites, our excesses.

"So there I was surrounded by all these brownies and cakes and ice cream and champagne. And I'm explaining to Karen why I can't eat these things." Lisa is telling me about her cousin's wedding shower. It has become a familiar story, deprivation in the midst of abundance.

We're in my sunny, glassed-in kitchen nook. The sharp smell of garlic-broccoli soup steams our faces. Rye crackers, unleavened. Healthy food, no yeast, no sugar.

"People always think I'm anorexic if I don't explain. And Karen says, 'Oh, Renee has candida, too.' And she points across the room to one of her friends, this really thin woman in dark glasses.

"I was so excited to find someone else. I went up to her and said, 'How are you handling it? What can you eat? Is it hard when you go out?' We were comparing diets and what kind of acidophilus we take." Animated, Lisa's face holds color under a dusting of brown eyeshadow and mulberry-slicked lips. It's a relief to see her spirits back. She's adjusting, I think, and then recoil at the thought. Adjusting? All of us adjusting to pollution, violation, invasion, illness?

"Renee got so sick she had to be hospitalized. She thought she had pneumonia until they finally diagnosed her. It would have been really dangerous if it had gone on." I see a flicker of fear in Lisa's eyes. At least she never became that ill.

"And when I was complaining about the diet, Renee said, 'Well, you'll get used to it.'"

Necessary adaptation. So here we are. With our broccoli soup. With our brain fog and swollen glands and sore throats. Though Lisa's illness, hopefully, will never be as severe as that of a person with CFS, we understand each other in a new way, strange allies in illness, bonded in a way we would not have chosen—and in another way I don't as yet suspect.

It will be several more years before I page through enough research to connect my chronic sore throat to yeast. When I ask my physician if the white coating on my throat could be thrush, he takes a quick look and says no. I insist he take a culture, which comes back negative. It will be several more years before I ask another physician to take a look at those test results, and discover that the doctor had ordered a test for strep, not yeast. Even my acupuncturist, inexplicably, crinkles her nose and pronounces my throat is not colonized by yeast. She never mentions diet. Going on my own hunch, in the spring of 2001 I will put myself on an antiyeast diet, with significant reductions in my sore throat, brain fog, allergies, and PMS.

Are Lisa and I bonded, too, with countless others, all those whose immune systems are under siege? What medical specialty will take up these questions? Who will count us, collect the data about our lives? Who will be independent enough to address the questions that may challenge the basis of our commercial culture and consumption patterns? The small number of clinicians or researchers who take seriously illnesses such as candida, CFIDS, MCS, or fibromyalgia are often marginalized by their peers. The conservatism and caution of the mainstream scientific and medical community when pressed to examine the validity and implications of these illnesses are ironic indeed. The time is over for restraint.

17

Limbo

We had all, in our ways, been undermined by sickness—had lost the careless boldness, the freedom of the well. We could not be thrown back into the world straight-away. We had to have an in-between—existential as well as medical, a place where we could live a limited existence—limited and protected, not too demanding—a limited, but steadily enlarging, existence—until we were ready to re-enter the great world.

—Oliver Sacks, *A Leg to Stand On*

August 1999

Through the years of my illness I have come to a grudging truce with patience, which is not one of my virtues. I haven't learned patience. Rather, I don't have the luxury of impatience. My life, my days, my healing unfold with a languor and steadiness that won't be rushed. I can't escape the patience of the body, the pace that controls and regulates my evolving recovery. I can be impatient, but like pressing my foot against the floorboards when I'm in the passenger seat, it won't do any good and, in fact, might slow my progress further.

I respect this steady patience that is larger than myself. I have to. Yet I value impatience for its desire, its signal that I'm ready to start again, to rebound, to go on. I value impatience for its assertion in the face of obstacle, its persistence, its yesness. Desire itself, for renewal, for the energy to carry on, fortifies. It becomes a substitute for experience, for what has been lost. Desire is what I still have.

I never imagined that after four years of slow recovery I would still view my world largely through a bedroom window, still feel a foreigner to the world. I'm stunned that I find myself among the housebound, able to walk on average four to six blocks, that I still have days when I'm too weak to walk more than a couple of houses up the street. My early imaginings that this illness was a temporary setback seem hopelessly naive. Last year, besides various appointments—acupuncturist, dentist, haircut—I went out to lunch once, shopping twice. One hour, back home. I would stand in a store stupefied by the density of color and chrome, harsh light, booming sound track as if I spun dizzily, the world a streaked blur. I practiced speed shopping at its most befuddled—grab a sweater, anything that looked passable, pay and get out. Back to catalogues for the rest of the year. Fortunately, the ill don't need to be fashion mavens.

But this year, as every year, I'm a bit stronger, more clearheaded, and as the summer heat turns the upstairs bedroom breathlessly hot, I'm itching to get out. So when my sister Laura calls from Seattle to announce she is getting married, my mind leaps with the idea: I will shop for a gift for her. Instantly I know I have to do this. I know what I want to get her and where I want to go. A platter from Sur La Table on Fourth Street. I could use a catalogue, could go in with another sister and let her do the shopping, but I want to do this, in no small part because of what Laura is doing for me. She's having the wedding in Berkeley, five minutes from my home.

My eyes fill with tears when she tells me the ceremony will be at the Claremont Hotel in the afternoon, perfect for me. A wedding in the Bay Area will be easier for all the sisters, aunts, uncles, and cousins spread around California to attend, but I know Laura is bringing the wedding down south to accommodate me, too. She wants all her sisters at her wedding. I am moved by her caring and love, like that of all my family, which has been there throughout my illness. Her voice chimes with energy. It's summer, the day is warm as a yeasty kitchen. At this moment I feel a crest of possibility, the way life comes at you in waves, its marvelous ability to expand. This wedding gift has the specter of a challenge. I will do it.

One morning in August I wake from a good night's sleep, feeling up to a short venture into the world. Bill can take a break from work this afternoon. This is the day to shop. After lunch, he stands in the door to our bedroom expectantly, his face tightened into an expression I've learned to decipher as a mix of hope and apprehension. He's still burdened by responsibility for me—will I be OK, is this a good idea?—but I know he feels as pleased as I do that we've reached this point, that shopping is even a possibility.

We climb in the car. In moments I'm transported from my bubble of calm to teeming commotion as we slice through neighborhoods, streets stacked one after another in huge blocks, a busy, intricate world that has been going on without me, trucks, bicycles, creosote roofs, boom boxes.

The release from stillness and solitude is startling. Bill drops me off while he goes to park, and I stand on the sidewalk like a tourist, someone from another country, taking in the cacophony, the high, reverberating blend of cars and shouts, a multitude of conversations and footsteps, wind, the distant freeway, doors opening. The world is so insistently vocal. A couple years ago my virally impaired brain could not have tolerated such overwhelming busyness and confusion. Today I can, for a short while.

Standing on Fourth Street, an upscale stretch of boutiques and restaurants in a former industrial area of the Berkeley flatlands, I take in a world transfigured in my absence. This is where the trendy shops have moved to get away from the homeless on Shattuck Avenue and the punks and students on Telegraph. Elegant housewares, garden shops, angled bookstores, Southwestern pink adobe walls, sidewalk benches, and tasteful window displays—the whole place blinding in its bustle and polish.

The glaring light of day on a city street transforms me, too. I'm suddenly ordinary, like everyone else, my infected, struggling body unseen, vanished in this landscape. Being invisible is invigorating, a reprieve. It brings alive that remarkable feeling of inhabiting a well body, of being once again an old self—wearing a teal blouse, earrings—that has felt so lost and distant. Energized, I want to step into all the shops, just to see them, to soak in this display of color, scents, and visual luxury.

When Bill joins me, I pull him into a small haberdashery, a perfumy rush of lilac and rose assailing us. The room is awash in lace, doilies, wooden crates spilling chalky soaps, pink and violet, creamy quilted bed jackets with silky ribbons, tiny satin pillows, baskets, floral wall hangings. The undiluted concentration of kitsch is like breaking a fast with a gravy-laden, sugar-rich smorgasbord. I'm awed by the sheer volume of *things,* the enormity of our imagination and appetites. The world has not stopped wanting in my absence. Wanting things of questionable taste, uncertain utility. But wanting. This, I understand. I have deprivation lust, where anything new and different looks beautiful, desirable, even the tacky, overwrought, and absurd. I finger the fine filigreed edge of crocheted potholders, trace cupids and hearts on a pink decoupage photo album. I love these things, love their sheer voluptuousness.

Bill scrunches his face. He hates this saccharine curlicue overload. I shouldn't squander my stock of energy here anyway.

Next door we're drawn into an Italian delicatessen, with its own wave of heady scent, crusty bread and brined olives, sharp cheeses, a salty thickness to the air. How odd to think it has been years since I've seen a refrigerated case of salads bathed in frosty light, an extravaganza of peppers, feta, and oil-drenched pasta. Bill buys a slice of focaccia, heavy and rich with rosemary. This simple gesture delights me, walking out with a handful of greasy warmth, biting into it.

Up the street I spy a women's clothing store. "How often do I shop? Let's take advantage."

Bill hesitates. "Are you sure?"

"I can last ten minutes."

The carpeted room is tastefully sparse, low racks and chrome. I grab a dusty-pink crinkle blouse, fumble with buttons in a curtained dressing room. Moments later I'm chatting with the salesclerk as she rings up my purchase. Such an ordinary encounter. I'm impersonating someone I used to be, making animated small talk, calling up the automatic mannerisms of stores, all the while feeling a detached awe that I'm actually doing this, and aware of the effort. My identity teeters briefly toward normalcy, an old self is warmed and set in motion. I recognize this self that shops and chitchats. And I recognize the schizophrenic tug between selves, one wired for public presentation, the other frayed and fizzled, circuits stormy with overload.

My brain is going groggy, that confused vibrating starting in my head, as if I'm inside a jukebox. Outside, package under my arm, that familiar heaviness weights my limbs. Crowds at cafe tables, languid and sun-washed, come at me like isolated still shots in an echoing haze. Women in tank tops and jeans, rocking a stroller with one hand, heads thrown back in laughter, unperturbed by the thrum and commotion of the street. Couples leaning intently toward each other, a leather jacket stretched over a lap. The street dissolves into a pinwheel of motion and noise, and the painful reality penetrates: that life they're enjoying—easy banter and camaraderie, a simple moment in a busy day—is not mine.

I'm fading fast. We make it to the kitchen store, and again I'm struck by the profusion, the astounding number of things to absorb, the sheer volume of things we think we need: egg beaters, spatulas, glinting stainless steel, painted pottery, stacks of towels and wooden chopping blocks, fluted cake pans, wire mesh displays strung with gadgets, a carousel of glossy colors and glitter that pulses around me. What a contrast to the rarefied, simplified life of illness, where slippers, sweats, and a few books are enough.

Bill can tell I'm too weak to go wandering around the store, up and down aisles. "You stay here. I'll scout the platters."

"Thank you, thank you."

In minutes he's back. There are only two platters. He leads me to them. We eliminate the first one quickly, a fruit-painted bowl, too workaday. But the second is perfect, a sage and mushroom oval with brushstroke paintings of artichokes and fennel. Eureka! Quickly Bill gives the saleswoman his credit card, saying we'll call later with the mailing information, and we're out of there. He heads up the street for the car while I sag on a sidewalk bench, bundling away a few last details—the slick yellow boat varnish on the teak bench, the pigtails on a young girl sticking up like fountains—bringing what is distant and fleeting into me. I shut my eyes as we drive home, worn out, the streets a steady huff and rattle like old machinery.

From lattes and shops I'm whisked back to another sort of simple dailiness—manuscripts, dishes, and naps. Bill disappears into his office. I fill my water glass, drop my city clothes on the floor, and slip into bed. Soft mattress, smooth sheets. It's a relief to collapse into my familiar room, to be the person I am. A dull ache runs through my muscles, and my whole body seems to vibrate with a jangly residual that lasts for hours after I've been out, like an afterimage that stays on the retina.

"The world is too much with us," Wordsworth famously lamented. There comes a point in exhaustion when I don't want anything but rest. The voluminous world seems almost grotesque in its babel and din. I want nothing but my calm, skylit room, the window-framed branches of Japanese maple, patterned against a wash of blue. I can feel the missing limb of my life, its residual pain, but it's hard to find appeal in that busyness when a cottony fog swaddles my brain and a sandbag-heavy fatigue pulls me down. The forced retreat of illness can bring a bitter-sweet relief. With surrender comes a strange contentment, a placidity fuller than the simple relaxation after a busy day. It is much more pro-found, a collapsing into the self that is unmuscular and limp, and in some way deeply soothing. When I think of all those years I heaved my ill body forward into work or a night out, rest seems a prized state. A part of me has longed for the inner balance that comes with this realign-ment with the needs of my body.

If this makes seclusion sound pleasant or easy, it's not. I chafe every day. The desire for that former self, that life of conferences, parties, and hikes, fades in and out like a play of shadows, but doesn't ever disap-pear. I rest and rest, and then that other voice tunnels up, "The world is not with us enough." This was poet Denise Levertov's crisp reply to Wordsworth, almost two centuries later. Their cross-century conversa-tion concerned the origins and nature of poetry (Does the bustling city, the material world, deaden or drive poetic emotion and perception?), not the dilemma of a shut-in, but for me their words carry an uncanny resonance. Poets say more than they know. The world is too much with me. The world is not enough with me.

Like Levertov, I crave the everyday encounter with a vibrant urban world. It's my brain that is Wordsworthian, my compromised, strug-gling brain that demands the romantic view: nature as wellspring and tranquil solace. Fitting, I think, since the romantics elevated perception and recognized its power, for better or worse, to shape one's sense of the world. If my brain says the world is exhausting and depleting, then it is.

To restore his soul, Wordsworth had his beloved Lake District, his brooks and lanes, periwinkle and woodsorrel. I have my windowed view, the shaggy open arms of Monterey pine. Hummingbirds dart by, clouds gather and clear. Nature from a distance, tamed and framed. An urban idea of the natural world, in small parcels, against a background of grinding truck gears and distant, metallic clanging.

"Are you all better?" a friend asked over the phone. I hadn't spoken to her in a couple of years; I'd called to invite her over, to reconnect.

All better? I felt that familiar gulf—a chasm, really—that sense of opaque, dense distance between myself and others, between my experience and the ideas people carry around about this thing called "chronic fatigue syndrome."

"Better. I'm better."

The abstractions of language fail me, fail us. Other people's concept of better doesn't float in the same realm as mine. If I say I'm better they think I must be out and about, no longer home in bed. To me, better means this: In year three, on my absolute best day, I managed to walk eight blocks, a half mile, but I couldn't repeat this distance again, and the next few days I was unable to walk at all. In year four, this year, I managed to walk eight blocks five or six times, and once I could do it two days in a row. No healthy person imagines the process of regaining strength—and this is only one measure of my illness's severity—in such minute, glacial increments.

I wanted to be positive with my friend, but the fact is, people who are ill as long as I have been don't get all better. Once, when I was trying to explain to an aunt and uncle on the phone that I'm probably not going to make a full recovery—I was struggling to accept this fact myself—they leapt in with "Oh, you never know!" As if I'm not being positive enough, losing faith. My cheery family.

The question of recovery looms large over the CFIDS community. Few prognosis studies have been done, and those that have been conducted have been too small to be considered statistically valid. A 1997 article in the *Quarterly Journal of Medicine* reviewed a number of outcome studies and concluded that fewer than 10 percent of CFIDS patients made a substantial recovery, though a majority showed improvement after one-and-a-half to four years. One-fourth to one-third reported that their symptoms became worse over time.[1] A small 1999 follow-up study of twenty-three patients with severe CFIDS showed that after four years only one had fully recovered, or 4 percent.[2] Nine of these patients, or 39 percent, experienced improvement. A larger study published in 2003 found that about 10 percent of patients achieve complete remission.[3] A 2005 paper that analyzed multiple studies examining patient improvement over time put the median rate for full recovery at 7 percent and for showing improvement at 39.5 percent.[4]

Generally, the figure of 4 to 12 percent is used for full recovery. The greatest chance for recovery is believed to be in the first two to six years of illness. After this, the chances of a complete recovery appear to be slim. Anecdotally, no one I know has ever heard of someone ill longer than fifteen years who recovers fully. While many people appear to slowly improve, some people neither get better nor worse, and some worsen over time.

A follow-up study by Dr. David Bell of his pediatric patients who had been part of the cluster outbreak in Lyndonville, New York, in the mid-1980s, showed that thirteen years later 80 percent of patients had improved.[5] (Interestingly, Dr. Paul Cheney and others have noted that pediatric patients have a higher rate of improvement and recovery than do adults.[6]) However, when Dr. Bell asked more detailed questions about their functional abilities, more than half of those who labeled themselves improved said lingering symptoms limited their activity. They had adopted lifestyle changes such as activity reduction and flexible schedules in order to cope with their illness. Those who had been most severely ill, missing the most school or showing the most cognitive difficulty, had the poorest outcome.

Dr. Bell's study, which looked at only thirty-five children, underscores that the use of the term "recovered" must be provisional and tempered by a full understanding of the level of accommodation that enables a person to feel better, and an understanding that a person's condition can change over time. My own experience is telling: Had I been questioned in 1989, nine years after the onset of my illness, I would have said I was largely recovered, though I still had lingering fatigue. Yet in 1995 I was the sickest I'd ever been.

In one of the few studies of long-duration patients, those ill more than ten years, Dr. Fred Friedberg found that of 298 patients, 128 were worsening, 70 improving, and the rest staying the same.[7] Comparing the long-duration group (median eighteen years) to a short-duration group (median three years), he found that the long-term sufferers experienced greater severity of symptoms, particularly cognitive difficulties, such as memory and concentration impairment, word-finding difficulty, and confusion. They also showed onset at a younger age (28.1 years versus 42.2 years), a higher incidence of infection with mononucleosis and human herpesvirus 1 and 2, and a higher incidence of a comorbid condition, such as fibromyalgia, chronic sinus infections, thyroid problems, or asthma. Fully 83.3 percent of long-term sufferers were unable to work, compared to 51.5 percent of those with short-duration illness.

Clearly, much more research is needed. Funding to support larger, more rigorously designed studies must be a priority if we are to better understand the illness course and to discover causes, treatments, and a cure. At this point, predicting who will recover and when remains impossible. These and many other questions remain unanswered.

18

Returning

When liberation from the hospital comes, as welcome as it is, one's
real trouble begins: the trouble of remaking a sense of purpose as the
world demands.

                    —Arthur W. Frank, *The Wounded Storyteller*

October 1999

Illness is often thought of as a journey. I think of it as an outpost,
a place of remove. Its loneliness challenges, but this same isolation is a buffer. There's plenty of time to think, to reevaluate, make new
covenants with the self about habits, priorities, work, relationships. In a
sense it's the easy place to be because it's a place of imagining. The
return is the hard part. I face the task of making real what has been
imagined, constructing a life that supports health.

I no longer look like the person in that photo by the side of my bed,
that picture of Bill, Lisa, and me taken at a friend's wedding with our
wine glasses and gay smiles just months before I became so ill in the fall
of 1995. That photo was my marker in those terrible early months of illness, my placeholder, preserving an image of who I was and would be
again. It kept up my spirits, reassured me, gave me a goal and focus as I
healed: I would be that person again.

These days when I glance at that photo I see the distance between
that moment and now, between that person and who I have become.
Gazing at it I gaze into my past. I won't be that person again. I'm older,
more gray hair, more sags and bags in the expected places. Each step for-

ward as I heal over these months and years is a reclamation of some small sliver of my life, and a leaving behind. I won't be returned, none of us will.

Essayist Andre Aciman, eloquent chronicler of change and elision, observes in *False Papers,* "To measure time by how little we change is to find how little we've lived; but to measure time by how much we've lost is to wish we hadn't changed at all."[1] His circuitous thought mirrors the tangled inevitability of loss and change that winds through every breath, for me no different than for anyone.

In fact, the photo that preserved a self I wanted to recapture is itself misleading, the picture of health and carefree vitality it creates an illusion. I was not vibrant with health but quite ill at the moment the camera flashed, still recovering from a severe flare-up after a trip to Costa Rica three months earlier. In a sense, it is a picture of a person who didn't exist, and my clinging to that image an exercise in duplicity. Just months away from the collapse in the fall of 1995 that would change my life, I stood on a fragile precipice. I made it to the wedding, barely. When we pulled into the parking lot and saw how large the gardens were, I groaned. Could I walk from the parking lot to the grassy wedding site? Bill went ahead to check, leaving me in the car. Yes, he leaned his head in the window, it looked like a quarter-mile dirt road. I could manage.

I was thrilled to be celebrating with friends, to be out in the warm summer evening, to share in this most special moment. We snapped that photo under the shady pepper trees as the air rang with greetings and champagne fizz, in a moment of exhilaration. But after the ceremony, after grilled salmon and baby carrots, as the sun set and the dancing began, I was too exhausted to join in. We left, and I went home to bed. The self in that photo—bright, relaxed—the self I hoped to recover, was a publicly presented self, at odds with an inner reality. To hang on to that image is to hold to a dream of self. The crazy thing is, I still want that dream, just as then I still wanted those brief moments of celebration with friends. They were real, those moments, even if they floated on a deceptive surface.

Now I cling to them in memory, and in this way they're still mine, though the capacity of body, the image of health they stand for, eludes me. I'm still returning to that captured moment. I will continue to return, since I'm one of the lucky ones with this illness, among those who slowly get better.

I'm trying to return, though, not to a false moment, a dangerous illusion, but to a participation that can be sustained. If the sharp fracture with a previous life that took place that fall is to be redeemed, this is how. By building this new life on solid ground. By creating a life that supports healing.

I'm not sure what this means. It's not as if the architecture of my life will look any different or I will be miraculously transformed. Illness narratives are often cast as conversion narratives: A catastrophic event or upheaval forces reevaluation and change. A different person emerges from the scalding experience. To be converted means to be "turned around," to head in a new direction.

My life has indeed been turned around—and wrung inside out—but is the shift merely external, in my forced, homebound routine? Have I been turned around *inside*? I'm not so sure. As writer and Zen practitioner Scoop Nisker observes, people don't undergo temperament transplants. One CFIDS patient wrote about the value of preemptive rest, stopping for a short rest before you're exhausted. Sounds like a good idea. Have I done it even once? Make myself rest when I still have an ounce of energy? The new knowledge of the head doesn't so easily dislodge the lifelong, entrenched patterns of the body. On the other hand, of necessity, I go to bed early, eat my vegetables, let Bill run my errands. I like to think I'm better at stopping when I really need to, at asking for support, at accepting the necessity of a less active, though no less full, life. I like sociologist Kathy Charmaz's insight: "The problems with which ill people struggle are existential; their solutions are often organizational."[2]

To talk about returning suggests movement, packed bags, a destination reached. Yet I'm still lying in bed, still at home. No movement can be seen. I still have my leafy backyard view, that old Monterey pine, my skylights and white walls. I still have my routine: read client manuscripts in my bedroom in the morning; putter around the house, take a short walk, read and rest in the afternoon. Instead of movement there are simply moments, in the same place, when I can do something more easily than last year: walk eight blocks instead of six, read until four in the afternoon instead of three, on a good day. To see return I have to look at small routines, scan years. My return involves no geography but the self. It seems more of a stitching together, a repair job, a reappearance of someone familiar.

I am feeling more recognizable to myself these days, and to Bill. We have moments tinged with a precious normalcy. This morning I woke with an overpowering desire: I had to have pancakes. I had wakened from a food dream: an enticing platter of eggs, ham, applesauce, pastry, potatoes. I was starving, as I often am as soon as I wake. I had the urge to go out to Rick and Ann's, a nearby breakfast place that has luscious corn pancakes, broiled pork chops, and homemade cinnamon applesauce, but I knew that effort would be too much. Pancakes, though, I could do.

I stumbled downstairs in my nightgown, giddy with anticipation, and whipped up some light wheat-banana cakes, filling the air with a satisfying warm-bread smell. Bill and I stuffed them in our mouths standing at the stove, folding them in our hands with sour yogurt, feeling as if we'd stolen a Saturday morning in the middle of the week, a delicious way to start our workday. Eating them on impulse, savoring their doughy sweetness, was a victory. Anytime I can indulge, can have a brief moment that feels ordinary and fun, I feel how far I've come.

On a good day, those gray, fraught months start to seem distant, something I comment on to Bill over dinner. Remember when you had to help me walk across a room? When I was too ill to talk or read? I've moved away from that island of pain, dislocation, and isolation. I measure distance from a different perspective. Distance that once was the source of pain—my distance from a former life and from others—has become distance from a difficult time, and a measure of healing.

With time and improvement, my anger has diminished—anger at misunderstanding, at ignorant doctors, at Bill's confusion and distrust. Like healing, getting over anger is not something I can rush. It has its own time line of slow dissolution, and I often think of it as an organic process no different than the slow repair of cells that marks my recovery.

The slow repair of my relationship to Bill is another process that cannot be rushed. It happens, like pain itself, in small moments and daily acts. A moment in which he surprises me with a book he knows I've been wanting. Or when I smooth a dollop of lotion over the symmetrical curves of his back. Or when we get together with friends or family, something we're now able to do once a month or so. We see, more of the time anyway, that person we first fell in love with, or at least the older/newer version of that person.

There are other changes, ones more subtle than an altered routine or more carefully guarded rest time. My perspective has shifted. I see myself, more than I used to, as connected to that sweating suicidal man on the couch at a CFIDS support group years ago—not because I've ever been suicidal, but because I recognize the thin and precarious surface we glide along each day, and the ease with which an intact self can be shattered. I grasp with a visceral knowledge the vulnerability of the body and the self to loss and disruption, the way the self can be "unmade," as writer Elaine Scarry has said. Arthur Frank, a cancer survivor, describes how humbling is this new understanding: "The realization that obsessed me during chemotherapy was how easily every strength I thought I had could be reduced to weakness."[3]

At its worst, this frightening realization of the body's fragility makes me more anxious. At its best, it makes me a better listener to other people's stories of suffering, someone who won't turn away. It makes me better attuned to our common struggles, and better able to meet and appreciate each moment on the way. In this enhanced response, I can find, where there has often been distress, a glimmer of purpose and meaning.

Perhaps the most radical change is that I can no longer talk only about the public surface of my life. Illness forces a conversation about things we usually prefer to leave unspoken: intimate relationships, the body, pain. I'm not very good at this conversation; in fact, I'd rather not be having it at all. But without this discussion it would be too easy to revert to the old patterns, my own and our culture's, of soldiering on and ignoring weakness. We can't have the conversations we need—about medical research, public policy, environmental degradation—if we don't first talk about the ill body. And we can't talk about the ill body if we don't first see it.

It's unlikely there will be a conclusion to this story, an end, a point of saying, it's over. For me, CFIDS is an ongoing improvisation, though with a fairly well-anticipated trajectory: increasingly able to function like a more normal person, but never able to forget that I live in the land of the chronically ill, and that I cannot misstep. A pattern of ups and downs, exacerbations and rebounds, with a steady movement toward that place called "better."

EPILOGUE

Body of Knowledge

March 2005

The CFIDS landscape has changed significantly since I began scribbling notes for this book in the fall of 1997. In the mid-1990s, CFIDS research had stagnated, as many researchers, frustrated by the ineffective search for a viral agent, lost interest or questioned CFIDS's legitimacy. It was a time of discouragement and acrimony within the patient community. Breakthroughs, however, are often haphazard and come from the least expected places.

Who would have guessed that in 2002, the CDC would launch the most comprehensive and ambitious CFS research program ever, headed, even more astonishingly, by Dr. William Reeves, a onetime detractor. The result of a huge push from patient advocates, particularly the CFIDS Association of America, and the restoration of the $12.9 million the CDC misallocated in 1995–98, the research includes cutting-edge studies in microarray technology that could finally produce a diagnostic test for CFIDS. Federal funding for CFS research is still shamefully low given how serious and widespread this illness is, but the current federal effort is nonetheless significant. Other CDC goals are to understand whether CFS is one disease or many, to define the natural history and clinical presentation, to educate health-care providers, and to identify the pathophysiology, causal agents, and risk factors.

As the scientific community takes CFIDS more seriously, and as more people have witnessed or heard about the daily impact of this disease, credibility is increasing, gradually but noticeably. The public advocacy, the arguments and debates, the books and articles, and the steady traipsing of the ill into medical offices have had an impact. These days when I mention to someone that I have CFIDS, I sometimes get the response "Oh, that's hard," or "I'm sorry to hear that. I know how serious that can be." The relief I feel in those moments is like a long, slow exhale, a liberating release from isolation. The press no longer refers to the "yuppie flu." News stories today are more likely to portray CFIDS as the real, organic, and widespread illness it is. Most medical textbooks now include a section on CFS, and many physicians seem to be beyond expressing skepticism; instead, they are asking for information about what they can do to help their CFIDS patients.

In a major and surprising breakthrough in 2001, the CFIDS community gained a much-needed national spokesperson when CFIDS sufferer and writer Laura Hillenbrand's book *Seabiscuit: An American Legend* hit the best-seller lists. During the flurry of media attention that followed, news outlets were quick to pick up on the story within a story: Ms. Hillenbrand's struggle to write a book while battling CFIDS presented an uncanny mirror to Seabiscuit's underdog fight, with a battered jockey and down-and-out trainer, to race against and defeat the great War Admiral.

Ms. Hillenbrand gave over three hundred interviews to print and electronic media—by phone or on camera only if the interviewer came to her home—detailing her devastating illness along with the Seabiscuit saga, and bringing the day-to-day reality of this disease to life for millions. I had the thrill, along with thousands of others with CFIDS, of watching ABC and NBC declare on their national news broadcasts, as a lead-in to interviewing Ms. Hillenbrand, that CFS was a serious and debilitating illness that could last for years. In July of 2003, that flagship of magazines, *The New Yorker,* printed Ms. Hillenbrand's chilling personal story. More than a few friends e-mailed me after reading the article or hearing Ms. Hillenbrand speak, clearly impressed with the severe vision she gave of this illness.

The appalling fact remains, though, that it has taken more than twenty years and a rebellious movement by patients and lay advocates, pushing against entrenched scientific thinking, to force a more serious look at this disease. Doctors may give lip service to the medical school aphorism "Half of what we teach you is wrong; unfortunately, we don't know which half," but medical culture continues to discourage any challenge to accepted medical practice. With the benefit of hindsight, we now know that as the CDC first confronted this illness in the mid-1980s, "Key decisions regarding the name, case definition, epidemiology and treatment were made . . . within a sociopolitical context in which CFS was assumed to be a psychologically-based problem."[1] If you don't believe an illness is genuine, you're not going to allocate funds for research, and as Dr. Leonard Jason says, "If you underfund [research], you're not going to get the type of science that's needed. . . . In 1984 through '88 a series of mistakes were made that ended up producing a case definition that was problematic, epidemiology that was flawed, and etiological attributions ["it's all in your head"] that were inaccurate."[2] These mistakes, along with a terrible, trivializing name, hampered medical practice and had a profound negative impact on patient experience for the next two decades.

For all the recent advances, the cause and pathophysiology of CFIDS remain unclear, the research continues to be underfunded, and an estimated 83–90 percent of people with this illness are undiagnosed. Though the personal and economic costs of CFS are huge—in the United States, an estimated $9.1 billion a year in lost productivity, not counting medical costs and disability benefits—many in the medical community, the media, and the public at large remain uninformed about CFS's impact.[3] I have yet to find a doctor at my HMO (the largest in California) who knows enough about this illness to be able to assist in my care.[4] A 2001 survey of physicians conducted by the CFIDS Association revealed that 92 percent felt more professional education about CFS was needed.[5] Western medical practice is not organized to provide the holistic, patient-centered, interdisciplinary approach to disease that CFS and other complex chronic illnesses require. The voice of the body continues to be devalued if it conflicts with established medical thinking. Though some people feel alternative remedies have helped them improve, for most, treatment remains limited to management of symptoms. And as we enter a time of record deficits and terrorism, SARS and bird flu, the federal budget for CFIDS, from the CDC and NIH, is once again shrinking.

Because fiscal year 2005 is the last year that the CDC is receiving "payback" funds for CFS research, to make up for the CFS funds diverted to other projects in 1995–98, without a significantly increased commitment, CDC funding will drop. NIH funding is also on the decline. Despite the fact that Congress has asked the NIH since 1990 to expand its CFS studies, NIH funding for CFS stagnated between fiscal years 1999 and 2003, a period during which the NIH budget grew by 76 percent.[6]

Most devastating has been the closure in 2003 of three NIH-funded CFS Cooperative Research Centers—at the University of Miami, the University of Washington, and the University of Medicine and Dentistry of New Jersey—that were established to encourage multidisciplinary collaborations, train young investigators, and provide an infrastructure for ongoing research. Since NIH funding confers legitimacy and prestige and serves to attract young scientists to a particular field, this loss of funding is a great threat to ongoing CFIDS research. Says the recently married Kim Kenney McCleary, "Without a critical mass of investigators, it will be many more years before we have effective treatments and reliable diagnostics."[7] The axiom remains true: much has been accomplished, but much more remains to be done.

As for me, my slow slog toward recovery continues.

In 2000, five years after my collapse in the fall of 1995, I started showing up at one or two parties a year, moments of pure delight. And Bill and I finally managed a weekend away, an hour's drive north to an Italianate B & B in Stinson Beach, where I walked a third of a mile two days in a row and relished the sea view. It took a mere week to recover.

After six years I had the thrill of walking my daughter down the aisle and dancing at her wedding, lingering under the stars till ten in the evening. Two months to recover, but a lifetime of gratitude that I could thoroughly enjoy that day.

After seven years, on a good day, I could edit client manuscripts for three hours in the morning, do some light reading lying down, and putter around the house for a few hours more. I could head out the door for my walk, still at six to eight blocks, but faster and more consistently. (Still plenty of days, though, when I was flared and could only work an hour and a half or walk half a block.)

After eight years, my sore throats began getting worse. I couldn't talk for four months out of the year, and had to limit my talking for another four. But that June of 2003, after a nearly sleepless night and jumping with excitement, Bill and I raced over to Kaiser Hospital in San Francisco to hold in our arms our new grandson, Zane David, 7 lb., 12 oz. Six weeks to recover, but to have held Zane in his first hours, to have shared that moment with his exhausted and euphoric parents, was an unsurpassed victory.

In 2004, after nine years, on a good day going out to lunch nearby had become pretty easy, as had the occasional short shopping trip or errand. I was sometimes active around the house, doing dishes or watering, as late as seven in the evening.

Today in 2005, as I approach the ten-year mark, it's clear that over the last couple of years I've shifted into that third phase of illness that Dr. Paul Cheney calls the "dynamic injury phase." My body still doesn't work right, my sore throats persist, but I'm no longer fully housebound and my brain fog and pain have receded to a low-moderate level. My functioning is limited—two short trips out of the house a week, fifteen to twenty hours of work a week, at home, and four to eight blocks of walking a day—but I have a life, in fact, a good one. Bill and I have been talking about a trip to the mountains, and the other evening he riffled through his files to find maps of the Sierra foothills, then spread them on the bed. When I traced my finger along the red curving line from the Bay Area to the vacation spot we'd chosen, it seemed a remarkable place to go.

Afterword

Nancy Klimas, M.D.,
University of Miami School of Medicine

When people question the legitimacy of chronic fatigue syndrome, or suggest it is a poorly understood illness, I always say we know a great deal about chronic fatigue syndrome. CFS has identifiable biologic underpinnings. Research has documented a number of underlying pathophysiologic processes involving the brain, the immune system, the neuroendocrine system, and the autonomic nervous system. The immune system is malfunctioning in two ways. It's chronically activated, so that the cytokines, the chemicals the immune system makes to stimulate immune responses, are elevated, producing many of the symptoms that CFS patients experience: achiness, brain fog, exhaustion. And the cells that are key to combating or suppressing viral infections are not working as well as they should. The neuroendocrine system is also functioning poorly, producing subtle hormonal imbalances. If you measure any particular hormone in a person with CFS, you will probably find that hormone in the normal range. But if you look at all the hormones as a group, you see that they cluster in the lowest range of normal as compared to controls.

The autonomic nervous system (ANS) is another key player in CFS. We learned a lot about the ANS in the mid- and late 1990s, starting with the work of Peter Rowe at Johns Hopkins University. He and his colleagues demonstrated that about 60 percent of CFS patients have a problem with regulation of blood pressure. In normal controls, the change in blood pressure and pulse from lying to standing is minor, perhaps five points. A person with CFS can have a twenty- or thirty-point change. It's very dramatic. What's even more fascinating, studies here at the University of Miami have shown that such rapid blood pressure change triggers an immediate inflammatory immune response in which cytokines (chemical messengers) are released. This in turn triggers a relapse of the patient's CFS symptoms, the pain, the swollen lymph nodes, the sore throat. None of these symptoms sound like they should be tied to a blood pressure drop, but they are. If people have these daily triggering events because of a drop in blood pressure, they have daily inflammatory consequences.

Sleep is another key element in CFS. Patients seem to be trapped in a very light alpha-wave sleep, unable to get down into the deeper, restorative phases of sleep. These restorative phases are very important biologically, as this is when the neuropeptides and hormone systems reset themselves and establish a normal circadian rhythm. As a clinician who cares for CFS patients, I know that if and when I'm lucky enough to get the sleep cycle adjusted, I almost always have a much healthier patient. While a number of current studies are trying to sort out the nature of the nonrestorative sleep cycle, we don't have nearly enough sleep experts looking at the problem of nonrestorative sleep in CFS.

We know that as a result of these biologic abnormalities, people with CFS can be seriously disabled. Dr. William Reeves and his team at the CDC have conducted research demonstrating that those with CFS can be as severely impaired as patients with congestive heart failure or chronic obstructive pulmonary disease (COPD). I have patients who are bedbound or housebound, and who are so profoundly ill I've only been able to see them by making house calls. I've had patients come into my clinic on stretchers or in wheelchairs. On the other end of the spectrum, I have patients who still work full-time, though they can only do that by sacrificing other parts of their lives. People with CFS find their work, social, recreational, and family lives restricted in significant ways. The average annual loss in household income due to CFS is estimated at

$20,000, half the average household income. That adds up to an enormous personal economic loss over the years, as well as a huge loss in tax revenue, an increased burden on the health-care system, and other societal costs. And dollar amounts can't begin to capture the emotional toll on individuals and families.

Sometimes people ask, "Is CFS an immune disorder? Is it a brain disease? Is it a dysfunction of the endocrine system?" I say it's all of these things. These four systems—the brain, the immune system, the neuroendocrine system, and the autonomic nervous system—are all integrated. What's more, they are all directed by chemical mediators. They're all giving chemical signals to cells in other parts of the body to tell those cells what to do. The brain is telling the peripheral nervous system what to do. The endocrine system sends out hormones, chemicals that influence tissues far away from the initial site. Lymphocytes, cells in the immune system, have receptors for all the neurotransmitters produced by the brain, and the brain in turn has receptors for all the cytokines, the chemicals released by the immune system. So all these systems are communicating with and influencing each other. You can't separate them.

Yet scientists, working within their own disciplines, have tended to see CFS through a narrow lens, much like the story of the old blind men and the elephant. Three blind men come upon an elephant and are confused about what they've encountered. One grabs its tail, one its trunk, and one its leg. The one touching the leg says, "Oh, I know what this is. This is a tree." And the one holding the tail says, "Oh, I know what this is. This is a snake, right?" And so on. This is how we initially approached chronic fatigue syndrome. As the immunologist, I would say, "This is clearly an immune dysfunction state." And the endocrinologist comes up and says, "Oh no, it's the adrenal gland." And the person focused on the autonomic system says, "No, no, this is all about blood pressure. What are you guys talking about?" The truth is that CFS impacts all of these systems in profound ways, and these integrated systems cannot be pulled apart if we hope to understand this illness.

Another heated debate has been over whether or not CFS is a form of depression. One of the biological markers of depression is an enlarged adrenal gland and an increase in cortisol production. In CFS, the adrenal gland is smaller than normal and makes less cortisol than is normal. This and other studies of mood and CFS show that depression can't explain the symptoms of CFS. And yet, can mood be affected? Absolutely. More than half of CFS patients will develop a major depression in the course of the illness. But, more than half of multiple sclerosis patients develop major depression. More than half of lupus patients develop major depression. Many more than half of chronic renal patients on dialysis develop major depression. So would we reclassify all of those as psychiatric disorders? Of course not.

We're often so busy trying to separate brain from body, so concerned with trying to categorize a disease as either mental or physical, that we fail to focus on all the systemic connections. As a condition that affects multiple body systems, CFS makes us look at the interrelationship between brain and body, and among the various body systems. Increasingly, scientists are adopting a more multidisciplinary approach and promoting scientific exchange and collaboration. I think we're now finally interested in multidisciplinary work, and we now have the tools to do it. It's a real exciting time.

CFS is also a disease that gives us the opportunity to understand the way very subtle shifts in chemicals can affect health. Basically, in CFS a whole host of chemicals that are supposed to bring messages from site A to site B so that the body functions correctly are not working efficiently. The basic chemical and hormonal balance is disrupted in a subtle way. We don't see large, obvious disruptions as we might in other conditions. For instance, if your cortisol production were to go below a certain level, we'd recognize that condition as Addison's disease. The degree of hormonal disruption in CFS is more minute, but still has an enormous impact on physical and mental functioning. Understanding the body on this finely tuned level is key to understanding health and disease, yet these kinds of subtle imbalances have not been a significant focus of research. The importance of this focus is by no means confined to CFS. The discoveries in our field should spur thinking and research in many other areas of medicine.

There are many medical disciplines in which a great deal is known. But we actually know very little about fatigue. What is fatigue? What causes it? What is the difference between mental fatigue and physical fatigue? And why can mental fatigue in CFS induce a physical fatigue, and vice versa? These are important questions that cross many fields. Yet we don't begin to understand the nature, the pathophysiology, of fatigue itself. We have many more questions than answers, and each question breeds more questions. There is a great deal to learn here. It's a fascinating area in which to do science.

Despite this fact, one of the problems with CFS research is that not enough scientists are interested. I believe one thing that prevents us from having as many scientists as we should in this area is that CFS is seen as predominantly a woman's disease. Plenty of studies have shown that a physician may respond differently to a patient based on that patient's gender. A man with symptoms of a heart attack, for instance, will be admitted to the cardiac care unit, while a woman with symptoms of a heart attack is likely to be sent home without a diagnostic study being ordered. Too often, if a woman walks into a doctor's office and says, "I feel profoundly fatigued, I hurt all over, and I can't do the things I used to be able to do," the doctor will say, "Buck up." Or he'll hand her a prescription for antidepressants.

The lack of credibility accorded this illness has been a key obstacle to understanding it. The patient has no credibility, the doctor who perceives the illness as real has no credibility, the researcher who's doing science in this area has a problem with credibility. The quality of CFS research in the medical literature has been criticized, in part because there are too many pilot-level studies that have yet to move into definitive and critical research. Yet the lack of more fully developed studies is in large part because research funding has been too limited. My job as a scientist is to build a credible set of studies in the medical literature to combat all the skepticism. But I can't do my job well unless there is a critical mass of science, unless there are many other scientists developing the kind of science that can't be ignored, in which the data supports the final conclusions.

I believe this area would be of far greater interest to scientists if there was a steady source of research dollars. Despite some recent efforts by the CDC, it is still very difficult to find funding in this area. We need to radically rework the funding strategies for CFS research, to draw more researchers to the field. There are no funded training grants in our field to help develop young investigators, no funded CFS Research Centers, since the NIH cut funding to these programs. There are no Centers of Excellence, a strategy used by the NIH for other illnesses to develop both clinical strength and research potential in a given field. There are no intramural researchers on the NIH campus working in this area, and there is no "home base" NIH institute that houses and funds CFS research. Rather, the illness has been assigned to the Office of Women's Health, which has not had a budget for extramural research, but works by trying to convince the funding institutes to find funds as meritorious individual protocols pass peer review. As exciting as the research gains have been, and they are exciting, it is tremendously discouraging to find that the United States, which leads the world in scientific funding and as a result scientific advances, is outspent by Japan in the field of CFS.

Clearly, in the area of CFS research and treatment, we have so many needs! There are at least 400,000 undiagnosed patients in the United States. Those "lucky" ones who do receive a diagnosis too often find that their medical team is uninformed and unhelpful, and their disability insurance carriers refuse to recognize their condition. The few informed physicians find themselves trying to care for patients without sufficient data to support their treatment decisions. When family members hear some doctors dismiss the illness and other practitioners suggest a variety of different treatments, they are baffled as to how best to help their loved one.

We need more work to understand the various biologic subgroups of CFS and to discover treatments that address the true biologic underpinnings of this illness. We need clinical trials data with patient groups that are large enough to answer questions about the efficacy and safety of various clinical approaches. We need to educate physicians and other health-care workers about this illness and keep at it until every doctor, nurse practitioner, and physician's assistant can quote the diagnostic criteria and treatment strategies. We need to educate the public and convince our legislators to authorize significant increases in CFS funding.

Urgent as these needs are, in 2005 we find funding for basic and clinical research dropping. We currently have less than a dozen NIH- or CDC-funded protocols. In the last four years, fewer than half the number of protocols were funded as compared to the four years preceding, and those preceding four years were already inadequately funded. And much of the work that is funded is the less expensive preliminary work that precedes fully developed, definitive studies. A Medline search reveals a flat line of scientific growth over the past fifteen years, with the same number of articles about CFS published roughly every five years since 1990. Yet the key research questions raised by CFS are basic to our understanding of human health and should easily draw the much-needed critical mass of investigators to the field.

It sounds discouraging, but despite these barriers, we have already learned a great deal about the biologic nature of CFS. New data from the CDC using information garnered from the human genome project suggests basic metabolic dysfunction and patterns of gene activation that are novel to this illness. These gene profiles may lead to targeted therapeutic interventions. With the latest prevalence data, which puts the number of people with CFS in the United States at 500,000 to 800,000, pharmaceutical companies are beginning to see CFS as a "market" and to express interest in clinical trials. The many patient advocates, researchers, and physicians who have dedicated their energies to understanding CFS and supporting and treating those who are ill remain committed. Many people are working to make a difference, and sometimes it is possible for one person to do something that makes a difference, too.

Dorothy Wall's story of her struggle with CFS is such an act. The picture she gives of daily life with CFS humanizes this illness, puts a face to the suffering, and shows how a person can maintain humor and dignity despite a culture of ignorance. Her experience is, sadly, all too typical, as she found herself terribly ill, misunderstood, and poorly treated by an uninformed medical establishment. Yet the personal courage and effort it took to write her book remind us of the human spirit that will not be defeated by ignorance.

Many other extraordinary folks are working to peel away the misconceptions surrounding this illness. Individual patients are writing letters to their legislators, and the legislators seem to be listening. National organizations, such as the CFIDS Association, fund-raise and support important projects: pilot money for research, lobbyists in Washington, conferences for patients and clinicians. There is much the individual person can do, and when we join in collective action that power is magnified.

Patients and those who love them often ask what they can do to help make a difference. CFS support groups are a great way to get connected and join in collective action. There are support groups in many communities across the country and around the globe. Some groups simply offer a safe environment in which to share experiences; others work to educate local physicians and media about the disease. Internet groups are another vital source of connection and activism. These groups can provide information and support for the homebound and those living in places that lack local patient networks, and they help keep patients abreast of research developments, and advocacy efforts and opportunities.

Many patients I've met over the years have found that becoming an advocate gives them a way to rise above the limits of illness. Whether that means raising funds for research, sharing articles about CFS with friends and health-care providers, or writing to members of Congress to urge increased research funding, the resulting feelings of empowerment can help replace the identity losses that often result from chronic illness. What we know about CFS today has been fueled by activism, and the important questions we have yet to answer warrant our sustained commitment to these efforts. I urge you to become involved.

APPENDIX

Resource List

Action for ME
Third Floor, Canningford House
38 Victoria Street
Bristol
BS1 6BY
Phone: Lo-call 0845 123 2380 or 0117 927 9551
Fax: 0117 927 9552
http://www.afme.org.uk

The UK's leading charity dedicated to improving the lives of people with ME. They provide information and support, and advocate for more research, and better treatments and services for people affected by ME.

American Association for Chronic Fatigue Syndrome (AACFS)
27 N. Wacker Drive, Suite 416
Chicago, IL 60606
Phone: (847) 258-7248
Fax: (847) 748-8288
http://www.aacfs.org

A nonprofit organization of research scientists, physicians, and other health-care professionals promoting scientific exchange and review of currrent clinical, research, and treatment ideas for CFS/FM.

American Chronic Pain Association
PO Box 850
Rocklin, CA 95677-0850
Phone: (800) 533-3231
http://www.theacpa.org

An organization dedicated to helping people better manage their pain and live more satisfying, productive lives.

Chronic Fatigue and Immune Dysfunction Syndrome Association of America
PO Box 220398
Charlotte, NC 28222-0398
Phone: (704) 365-2343
Fax: (704) 365-9755
http://www.cfids.org

The nation's leading charitable organization dedicated to conquering CFIDS by accelerating research, impacting public policy, and focusing attention on this serious public health concern.

ME Society of America
PO Box 44402
Shreveport, LA 71134
http://www.cfids-cab.org/MESA/

A research-information and advocacy group seeking to promote understanding of the disease known as myalgic encephalomyelitis (ME).

The National CFIDS Foundation
103 Aletha Road
Needham, MA 02492
Phone: (781) 449-3535
Fax: (781) 449-8606

http://www.ncf-net.org

An organization working to fund research and provide information, education, and support to people with CFIDS.

National Chronic Fatigue Syndrome and Fibromyalgia Association (NCFSFA)
PO Box 18426
Kansas City, MO 64133
(816) 313-2000
http://www.ncfsfa.org

An organization offering patient resources, physician resources, and research information.

National Fibromyalgia Association
2200 Glassell Street, Suite A
Orange, CA 92865
Phone: (714) 921-0150
Fax: (714) 921-6920
http://www.fmaware.org

A nonprofit organization dedicated to improving the quality of life for people with fibromyalgia by increasing the awareness of the public, media, government, and medical communities.

National Women's Health Resource Center
157 Broad Street, Suite 315
Red Bank, NJ 07701
Phone: (877) 986-9472
http://www.healthywomen.org

A nonprofit organization dedicated to helping women make informed decisions about their health and embrace healthy lifestyles. A national clearinghouse for women's health information.

Patient Alliance for Neuroendocrineimmune Disorders Organization for Research and Advocacy (PANDORA)
255 Alhambra Circle, Suite 715
Coral Gables, FL 33134
Phone: (954) 783-6771
Fax: (954) 785-9718
http://www.pandoranet.info

An organization raising awareness, providing support and educational resources, establishing partnerships, supporting research, encouraging creation of empowerment groups, and organizing conferences.

FEDERAL RESOURCES

Centers for Disease Control and Prevention
1600 Clifton Road
Atlanta, GA 30333
http://www.cdc.gov
CFS information: http://www.cdc.gov/ncidod/diseases/cfs/index.htm

One of the most up-to-date information Web sites on CFS, with many links to other organizations.

National Institutes of Health
Office of the Director
Building 1
1 Center Drive
Bethesda, MD 20892
http://www.nih.gov
CFS information: http://www4.od.nih.gov/orwh/

The NIH is the nation's medical research agency dedicated to improving health and saving lives.

OTHER INTERNET RESOURCES

About.com
http://chronicfatigue.about.com/od/cfsassociations/
 A list of British, Canadian, and U.S. resources, and many links.

CFIDS Emergency Relief Services, Inc.
http://www.cfidsers.org
 Helps CFIDS patients dealing with financial crisis.

CFIDS Grassroots Action Center
http://capwiz.com/cfids/home/
 Provides information and letter templates to communicate with members of Congress, public health officials, and the media about issues of concern to CFIDS activists.

CFIDS Link
http://www.cfids.org/subscribe.asp
 Free monthly e-newsletter distributed by the CFIDS Association of America.

Chronic Fatigue Syndrome Provider Education Project
http://www.cfids.org/treatcfs/
 A place for CFIDS care providers to learn about CFIDS and take a free online course.

Co-Cure
http://www.co-cure.org
 Co-Cure stands for "Cooperate and communicate for a cure." They work to further cooperative efforts towards finding the cure for the ill-

nesses commonly referred to as chronic fatigue syndrome (CFS) and fibromyalgia (FM).

Disinissues

http://groups.yahoo.com/group/Disinissues

Disinissues stands for DIS-ability IN-surance ISSUES. The organization provides information and advice about applying for, appealing denials of, and renewing Social Security Disability Insurance (SSDI), Supplemental Security Income (SSI), and private long-term disability insurance.

National Library of Medicine

http://www.nlm.nih.gov/medlineplus/chronicfatiguesyndrome.html

A searchable database of published medical literature called MEDLINE.

Pediatric Network for Chronic Fatigue Syndrome, Fibromyalgia, and Orthostatic Intolerance

http://www.pediatricnetwork.org

Established to help families and advocates connect.

Pro-Health

http://www.chronicfatiguesupport.com

For chronic fatigue syndrome and fibromyalgia news, support, and comprehensive nutritional solutions.

Notes

INTRODUCTION

1. Hillary Johnson, *Osler's Web: Inside the Labyrinth of the Chronic Fatigue Syndrome Epidemic* (New York: Crown Publishers, 1996), p. 10.

2. Ibid., pp. 31, 41.

3. Susan Sontag, *Illness as Metaphor and AIDS and Its Metaphors* (New York: Doubleday, 1989), p. 3.

4. Arthur Kleinman, M.D., *The Illness Narratives: Suffering, Healing, and the Human Condition* (New York: Basic Books, 1988), p. xiv.

5. George M. Beard, *A Practical Treatise on Nervous Exhaustion (Neurasthenia): Its Symptoms, Nature, Sequences, Treatment*, 2nd ed. (New York: William Wood & Co., 1880), p. vi, as cited in Susan E. Abbey, M.D., and Paul E. Garfinkel, M.D., "Neurasthenia and Chronic Fatigue Syndrome: The Role of Culture in the Making of a Diagnosis," *American Journal of Psychiatry* 148, no. 12 (December 1991): 1639.

6. Johnson, *Osler's Web*, p. 473.

7. See Dr. Cheney's presentation "New Insights into the Pathophysiology and Treatment of CFS," sponsored by the CFS/FM support group of Dallas–Fort Worth and videotaped in Dallas, Texas, October 2001.

8. David Morris, *Illness and Culture in the Postmodern Age* (Berkeley: University of California Press, 1998), p. 52.

9. Ibid., p. 70.

PROLOGUE

1. Dedra Buchwald et al., "A Chronic Illness Characterized by Fatigue, Neurologic and Immunologic Disorders, and Active Human Herpesvirus Type 6 Infection," *Annals of Internal Medicine* 116, no. 2 (January 15, 1992): 103. This illness cluster was later assumed to be CFIDS.

2. Ibid.

CHAPTER ONE

1. Juanne N. Clarke, Ph.D., "The Search for Legitimacy and the 'Expertization' of the Lay Person: The Case of Chronic Fatigue Syndrome," *Social Work in Health Care* 30, no. 3 (2000): 75. These 1997 figures actually showed an increase since 1993 in the belief that CFS has a psychiatric basis in depression or hysteria. In 1993 there were 145 articles on CFS listed on Medline, 21 percent attributing a psychiatric cause, 63 percent an organic cause, 16 percent other.

2. Elaine Showalter, *Hystories: Hysterical Epidemics and Modern Media* (New York: Columbia University Press, 1997). See in particular pp. 115–32. As many have noted, Showalter's ideas themselves fan the flames of antagonism and create a rather hysterical subculture of disbelief. The fact that so many people with CFIDS come to understand their illness, as I did, on the basis of media reports is due to the failure of Western medical doctors to recognize or understand this illness.

3. Johnson, *Osler's Web,* p. 645.

4. M. Reyes et al., "Prevalence and Incidence of Chronic Fatigue Syndrome in Wichita, Kansas," *Archives of Internal Medicine* 163, no. 13 (July 14, 2003): 1530–36.

5. In fact, Jason's research team had pressured the CDC to adopt many of the methods they were using, including random selection of a

community sample and medical examination of those with CFS symptoms, and the CDC did ultimately adopt these recommendations when conducting its 1998 study. Personal communication from Dr. Leonard Jason, October 2, 2003.

6. Leonard A. Jason, Ph.D., et al., "A Community-Based Study of Chronic Fatigue Syndrome," *Archives of Internal Medicine* 159, no. 18 (October 11, 1999): 2129–37. The DePaul University epidemiology study demolished a number of myths about CFS, revealing that CFS rates were higher among Latinos and African Americans than among whites, and that CFS rates among women ($^{522}/_{100,000}$) were higher than the rates for women with HIV ($^{125}/_{100,000}$), lung cancer ($^{43}/_{100,000}$), or breast cancer ($^{26}/_{100,000}$).

CHAPTER TWO

1. Katherine Anne Porter, *Pale Horse, Pale Rider* (New York: New American Library, 1967), p. 151.

2. Bettyann Holtzmann Kevles, *Naked to the Bone: Medical Imaging in the Twentieth Century* (New Brunswick, N.J.: Rutgers University Press, 1997), p. 275.

3. Robert Aronowitz, M.D., *Making Sense of Illness: Science, Society, and Disease* (Cambridge and New York: Cambridge University Press, 1998), p. 33.

4. Kevles, *Naked to the Bone*, p. 2.

5. Aronowitz, *Making Sense of Illness*, p. 5.

6. R. B. Schwartz et al., "SPECT Imaging of the Brain: Comparison of Findings in Patients with Chronic Fatigue Syndrome, AIDS Dementia Complex, and Major Unipolar Depression," *American Journal of Roentgenology* 162, no. 4 (April 1994): 943–51.

7. Mark Doty, *Heaven's Coast: A Memoir* (New York: HarperCollins, 1996), p. 252.

8. Schwartz, "SPECT Imaging of the Brain."

9. Phone interview with Dr. Anthony Komaroff, May 11, 2004.

10. Johnson, *Osler's Web,* p. 564.

11. For a detailed account of Hillary Johnson's investigation of the CDC funding scandal, see her book, *Osler's Web,* beginning with pp. 289 and 371.

12. "Audit of Costs Charged to the Chronic Fatigue Syndrome Program at the Centers for Disease Control and Prevention," June Gibbs Brown, Inspector General, Department of Health and Human Services, May 1999, p. 1.

13. "Public Health Service Funding, Chronic Fatigue Syndrome," document provided by the CFIDS Association of America.

14. Ibid.

15. "Estimates of Funding for Various Diseases, Conditions, Research Areas," online document, http://www.nih.gov/news/funding researchareas.htm.

16. Phone interview with Dr. David Bell, March 28, 2005. The chromium 51 technique was originally developed in the 1960s by a nuclear radiologist to diagnose congestive heart failure, a condition in which there is too much blood going to the heart.

17. Ibid.

18. D. Streeten and D. Bell, "Circulating Blood Volume in Chronic Fatigue Syndrome," *Journal of Chronic Fatigue Syndrome* 4, no. 1 (1998): 3–11. This study suggested that "a subnormal red blood cell mass and/or decreased circulating blood volume may well result in diminished cerebral blood flow with subnormal oxygen carrying capacity."

19. "Chronicle Q & A: Procrit Trial Focuses on Red Blood Cells," *The CFIDS Chronicle* 15, no. 4 (Fall 2002): 3.

20. The test Dr. Hurwitz and his associates used to measure both plasma volume and red blood cell volume is the dual tag blood volume test, the same test used by Dr. David Bell: one tag, I131, labels the plas-

ma albumin; the other tag, Cr51, labels the red blood cells. Interview with Dr. Barry Hurwitz, *The CFIDS Chronicle* 15, no. 4 (Fall 2002): 1. The results of the study are not known as of this writing, but Dr. Hurwitz asserts, "Even if Procrit does not improve CFIDS symptoms, the information we're collecting regarding circulatory functioning and immune system interactions in relation to fatigue will shed a great deal of light on some of the important disease pathophysiology." Ibid, p. 15.

21. Leonard A. Jason, Patricia A. Fennell, and Renee R. Taylor, eds., *A Handbook of Chronic Fatigue Syndrome* (Hoboken, N.J.: John Wiley and Sons, 2003), p. 565.

22. Personal communication from Peggy Munson, May 10, 2002.

23. Roy Porter, *The Greatest Benefit to Mankind: A Medical History of Humanity* (New York: W. W. Norton & Co., 1997), p. 679.

24. Ironically, the development of the social sciences in the twentieth century has meant that we have a much more sophisticated view of the patient as a complex subject today than we did in the nineteenth century. It's also the case that some health practitioners, such as Dr. Arthur Kleinman, have argued for the validity of a "lay perspective" that can be useful in understanding and diagnosing disease. But what we understand theoretically and what actually goes on in clinical practice are often two different things. Technological medicine and managed care continue to exert pressures on the medical encounter that work to marginalize the patient's subjective experience when it's not reinforced by objective findings and test results.

25. Dr. Robert Aronowitz gives an example of how medical focus has shifted from the patient to the pathology. "By midcentury [1900s], the authors of medical texts and research articles no longer showed much interest in the relationship of social and individual factors to the etiology and clinical course of angina pectoris that had been a major concern of clinicians and investigators writing about angina pectoris in the preceding decades. The narrowing of medical focus from the indi-

vidual to the coronary artery did not so much dismiss these relationships as reduce their centrality, especially to the heart specialist. Thus, descriptions of the typical angina pectoris patient and advice about how to use personal and social information to diagnose and manage the disease gradually disappeared from medical texts. Such descriptions and advice were replaced by more detailed anatomical and pathological information about CHD [coronary heart disease] and the role of objective signs (such as the white blood cell count and fever) and technology (use of the electrocardiogram) in diagnosis." Aronowitz, *Making Sense of Illness,* p. 123.

26. Porter, *The Greatest Benefit to Mankind,* p. 682.

27. Dr. Charles M. Poser, "The Differential Diagnosis of CFS and MS," *The CFS Research Review* 1, no. 4 (Fall 2000): 6. See also Johnson, *Osler's Web,* p. 215.

28. Johnson, *Osler's Web,* p. 368.

CHAPTER THREE

1. Elaine Scarry, *The Body in Pain: The Making and Unmaking of the World* (New York: Oxford University Press, 1985), p. 5.

2. Ibid., p. 4.

3. Anatole Broyard, "The Patient Examines the Doctor," in *Intoxicated by My Illness: And Other Writings on Life and Death,* comp. and ed. Alexandra Broyard (New York: Clarkson Potter, 1992), p. 53.

4. Sophocles, *Philoctetes,* trans. Judith Affleck (Cambridge: Cambridge University Press, 2001), p. 3.

5. Ibid., p. 57. Apparently, the original Greek is more complex. It's the translation that breaks down, compressing Philoctetes' shouts to an inexplicit A, a, a, a! Though universal, pain becomes, to this translator anyway, untranslatable.

CHAPTER FOUR

1. Dan Ouellette, "A Piano Genius Battles Back," *The San Francisco Examiner and Chronicle,* February 28, 1999.

2. Abstracts of papers presented at the Bi-Annual Research Conference of the American Association for Chronic Fatigue Syndrome (AACFS), October 10–11, 1998, Cambridge, Massachusetts, Name Change Session, presentation by Tom Hennessy, p. 15, online report, http://www.cfids-me.org/aacfs/change.html. For the name-change story, I drew on phone interviews and e-mail exchanges with Kim Kenney, Roger Burns, Peggy Munson, and Dr. Anthony Komaroff; many online documents; numerous issues of *The CFIDS Chronicle;* and Aronowitz, *Making Sense of Illness,* pp. 19–38, and Johnson, *Osler's Web.*

3. Johnson, *Osler's Web,* p. 228.

4. Aronowitz, *Making Sense of Illness,* p. 25.

5. Gary Holmes et al., "Chronic Fatigue Syndrome: A Working Case Definition," *Annals of Internal Medicine* 108, no. 3 (March 1988): 387–89.

6. Personal communication from Dr. Anthony Komaroff, May 16, 2004.

7. Leonard A. Jason, Renee R. Taylor, Sigita Plioplys, Zuzanna Stepanek, and Jennifer Shlaes, "Evaluating Attributions for an Illness Based upon the Name: Chronic Fatigue Syndrome, Myalgic Encephalopathy and Florence Nightingale Disease," *American Journal of Community Psychology* 30, no. 1 (February 2002): 140.

8. Ibid.

9. Online report, http://www.cfs-news.org/namebkgd.htm, January 17, 2001. Comments from Panelists at the Change the Name Forum of 1996, American Association for Chronic Fatigue Syndrome (AACFS) Conference, San Francisco, October 15, 1996.

10. *The CFIDS Chronicle,* Special Bulletin, November 1993.

11. Online document from RESCIND, http://www.geocities.com/capitolhill/4277, June 10, 2001, p. 9.

12. All quotes from Ms. Kenney and background information about the CFIDS Association's activities in the name-change effort are from phone interviews with Ms. Kenney, November 1, 2000, March 12, 2001, and May 10, 2002, and from various issues of *The CFIDS Chronicle,* particularly the November 1993 Special Bulletin.

13. *The CFIDS Chronicle,* Special Bulletin, November 1993, p. 14.

14. A Canadian educational/research foundation incorporated in 1988, named after Florence Nightingale, who suffered from an illness similar to CFIDS.

15. *The CFIDS Chronicle,* Special Bulletin, November 1993, p. 24.

16. Ibid., p. 9.

17. Ibid., p. 28.

18. Ibid., p. 29.

19. Though the 1994 Fukuda criteria were seen as an improvement over the 1988 Holmes criteria, investigators have continued to raise concerns about whether the Fukuda definition is specific and sensitive enough to exclude those with primarily psychiatric problems. "Even Fukuda, one of the primary authors of the U.S. case definition, has stated that the current CFS diagnostic criteria might not exclude people who have purely psychosocial stress, or many psychiatric reasons for their fatigue." Caroline King and Leonard A. Jason, "Improving the Diagnostic Criteria and Procedures for Chronic Fatigue Syndrome," *Biological Psychology* 68, no. 2 (February 2005), p. 88.

20. Phone interview with Roger Burns, April 26, 2001.

CHAPTER FIVE

1. John Bayley, *Elegy for Iris* (New York: Picador, 1999), p. 266.

2. Nicholas Regush, *The Virus Within: How Medical Detectives Are Tracking a Terrifying Virus That Hides in Almost All of Us* (New York: Penguin, 2001), p. 55. Regush cites the Centers for Disease Control's findings when they investigated the Lake Tahoe outbreak. "They discounted EBV because antibody levels of other common viruses, including CMV, herpes simplex 1 and 2, and even measles turned up higher than routine in those diagnosed with the illness."

3. Pasteur grudgingly acknowledged that the microbe wasn't the only culprit in disease. When Hermann Pidoux, a formidable medical figure of his time, insisted, "Disease exists within us, because of us, through us," advancing Bernard's argument, Pasteur replied, "This is true for certain diseases," then quickly added, "I do not think that it is true for all of them." Patrice Debre, *Louis Pasteur*, trans. Elborg Forster (Baltimore: The Johns Hopkins University Press, 1998), p. 261.

4. Johnson, *Osler's Web*, p. 132.

5. Buchwald, "A Chronic Illness Characterized by Fatigue, Neurologic and Immunologic Disorders, and Active Human Herpesvirus Type 6 Infection." The paper states, "Several groups of patients who had frequent close contact became ill within several months of each other: ten of thirty-one teachers at one local high school . . . ; five of twenty-eight teachers and three students at another local high school; three students and one teacher at a third high school; and eleven employees at a casino. The spouses or sexual contacts of six patients were similarly afflicted, and there were eight instances in which at least one parent and one child both had the illness" (p. 106).

6. Johnson, *Osler's Web*, pp. 5, 83, 226, 367.

7. David Perlman, "Fatigue Syndrome Still a Mystery," *The San Francisco Chronicle*, April 17, 1989.

8. Dr. Charles Lapp, director of the Hunter-Hopkins Center in Charlotte, North Carolina, mentioned to Dr. Leonard Jason that in Incline Village, just before the girls' basketball team got sick, the wood-

---

en floor had been redone; and in Raleigh, North Carolina, before the orchestra got sick, the floors were also redone. Personal correspondence from Dr. Leonard Jason, October 2, 2003.

9. Johnson, *Osler's Web,* p. 532.

10. "Is CFIDS Contagious?" *The CFIDS Chronicle* 9, no. 2 (Spring 1996): 7.

11. Ibid., p. 8. Asked for their opinions, other investigators echoed this response. A few suggested that while we can't be absolutely certain CFS is not contagious, it's unlikely that it is. Even Dr. Daniel Peterson of Incline Village, Nevada, hedged his response: "Certainly clusters of CFIDS such as occurred in Lake Tahoe, Yerington (NV), Placerville (CA), New York, North Carolina and many other areas suggest that a transmissible agent is at least a cofactor in the initiation of the disease process (in a susceptible host). As such, I concur with Ms. Johnson's postulate that CFIDS is a *potentially* contagious disorder" (emphasis mine). Ibid., pp. 7–9.

12. Ibid., p. 10.

13. *A Consensus Manual for the Primary Care and Management of Chronic Fatigue Syndrome,* online document prepared by the New Jersey Chronic Fatigue Association in conjunction with the New Jersey Department of Health and Senior Services (http://www.state.nj.us/ health/fhs/cfs_consensus_manual.pdf), p. 1.

14. Phone interview with Dr. David Bell, March 28, 2005.

15. Ibid. For further description of the two studies, see the CDC's online document "Chronic Fatigue Syndrome Program, Program Update, 2002–2003," http://www.cdc.gov/ncidod/diseases/cfs/program-updates/cfs-uptdate-031703.htm, pp. 5–6.

16. Dedra Buchwald et al., "A Twin Study of Chronic Fatigue," *Psychosomatic Medicine* 63, no. 6 (November/December 2001): 936–43.

CHAPTER SIX

1. Phone interview with Dr. Anthony Komaroff, May 10, 2004.

2. Natalie Angier, *Woman: An Intimate Geography* (New York: Houghton Mifflin Company, 1999), p. 283.

3. Carol Lee Flinders, *At the Root of This Longing: Reconciling a Spiritual Hunger and a Feminist Thirst* (San Francisco: HarperSanFrancisco, 1998), p. 138.

4. F. G. Gosling, *Before Freud: Neurasthenia and the American Medical Community, 1870–1910* (Chicago: University of Illinois Press, 1987), pp. 73–74.

5. Ibid., p. 74.

6. Ibid.

7. John H. Musser, M.D., and O. A. Kelly, M.D., eds., *A Handbook of Practical Treatment* (Philadelphia: W. B. Saunders Co., 1912), p. 868.

8. Charlotte Perkins Gilman, *The Living of Charlotte Perkins Gilman: An Autobiography* (Madison: University of Wisconsin Press, 1963), p. 95.

9. Ibid., p. 96.

10. Ibid.

11. Vicki Walker, "Working to Understand Why Activity Causes Relapse in CFIDS," *The CFIDS Chronicle* 17, no. 1 (Winter 2004): 9.

12. Patti Schmidt, "Should You Exercise?" *The CFIDS Chronicle* 11, no. 3 (May/June 1998): 18.

13. An Expert Medical Consensus Panel in Canada produced the first clinical case definition for ME/CFS (previous case definitions for CFS were research definitions) in 2003, saying of the previous American (Holmes 1988 and Fukuda 1994) case definitions, "The CDC definition, by singling out severe, prolonged fatigue as the sole major (compulsory) criterion, de-emphasized the importance of other cardinal symp-

toms, including post-exertional malaise, pain, sleep disturbances, and cognitive dysfunction." Bruce M. Carruthers, M.D., et al., "Myalgic Encephalomyelitis/Chronic Fatigue Syndrome: Clinical Working Case Definition, Diagnostic and Treatment Protocols," *Journal of Chronic Fatigue Syndrome* 11, no. 1 (2003): 9.

14. Schmidt, "Should You Exercise?" p. 18.

15. Gilman, *The Living of Charlotte Perkins Gilman*, p. 98. Just over a century later, best-selling author and CFIDS sufferer Laura Hillenbrand *(Seabiscuit: An American Legend)* would make a similar comment: "I know that some people are out there thinking, 'How sick can you be? You just wrote a 400-page book.'" Yet her illness was so severe as she worked that many days she could barely take a shower and often couldn't manage to leave her bedroom. "I have absolutely destroyed myself writing this book," she says of the effort. Hillenbrand quote from a sidebar entitled "Success and CFIDS: Fighting the Public Perception" accompanying an article by Mark Giuliucci, "A Matter of Dignity," *The CFIDS Chronicle* 14, no. 3 (Summer 2001): 3.

16. Tom Lutz, "Varieties of Medical Experience: Doctors and Patients, Psyche and Soma in America," in *Cultures of Neurasthenia from Beard to the First World War,* ed. Marijke Gijswijt-Hofstra and Roy Porter (Amsterdam/New York: Rodopi, 2001), p. 62.

CHAPTER SEVEN

1. Simon Wessely, "Old Wine in New Bottles: Neurasthenia and 'ME,'" *Psychological Medicine* 20, no. 1 (January 1990): 35–53; P. White, "Fatigue Syndrome: Neurasthenia Revived," *British Medical Journal,* no. 298 (1989): 1199–1200; D. B. Greenberg, "Neurasthenia in the 1980s: Chronic Mononucleosis, Chronic Fatigue Syndrome, and Anxiety and Depressive Disorders," *Psychosomatics* 31, no. 2 (1990): 129–37.

2. Margaret A. Cleaves, M.D., *The Autobiography Of A Neurasthene:*

As Told By One Of Them And Recorded By Margaret A. Cleaves, M.D.
(Boston: The Gorham Press, 1910), p. 18.

3. Ibid., p. 187.

4. Ibid., p. 70.

5. Ibid., pp. 64–65.

6. Ibid., pp. 19–20.

7. Ibid., p. 21.

8. D. Drummond, "The Mental Origin of Neurasthenia, and Its Bearing on Treatment," *British Medical Journal* 1907; ii: 1813–1816; J. Tinel, *Conceptions et Traitment des Etats Neurastheniques* (Paris: JB Balliere et fils, 1941), as cited in Simon Wessely et al., *Chronic Fatigue and Its Syndromes* (New York: Oxford University Press, 1998), pp. 106, 102.

9. Susan E. Abbey, M.D., and Paul E. Garfinkel, M.D., "Neurasthenia and Chronic Fatigue Syndrome: The Role of Culture in the Making of a Diagnosis," *American Journal of Psychiatry* 148, no. 12 (December 1991): 1638.

10. Edward Shorter, "Chronic Fatigue in Historical Perspective," in *Chronic Fatigue Syndrome,* Ciba Foundation Symposium 173 (Chichester, UK: Wiley, 1993), p. 9. Diagnoses have always been and continue to be influenced by physician belief. For example, in the nineteenth century, patients with similar complaints often received a different diagnosis depending on their class or gender. Men were more likely to be diagnosed as neurasthenic, women as hysterics. People of the lower classes were more likely to be labeled as insane and committed to an asylum, while someone of means, with the same symptoms, would be diagnosed as neurasthenic, a less stigmatizing label, and kept at home.

11. Ibid., p. 19, discussion comment by Dedra Buchwald.

12. Roy Porter, "Nervousness, Eighteenth and Nineteenth Century Style: From Luxury to Labour," in *Cultures of Neurasthenia from Beard to the First World War,* ed. Marijke Gijswijt-Hofstra and Roy Porter (Amsterdam/New York: Rodopi, 2001), p. 34. We can assume that class

bias was behind the equation of nervous ailments with the upper eche-lons of society, as was the case for George Beard's ideas about neuras-thenia. Cheyne's formulation was significant, however, in that it replaced humoralism with a more modern, mechanistic view of the body as a system of nerve pathways.

13. George Miller Beard, "Neurasthenia, or Nervous Exhaustion," *Boston Medical and Surgical Journal* 80 (1869): 245–59.

14. George M. Beard, *Sexual Neurasthenia (Nervous Exhaustion); Its Hygiene, Causes, Symptoms, and Treatment, with a Chapter on Diet for the Nervous,* ed. A. D. Rockwell (New York: 1884), p. 36, as cited in Barbara Sicherman, "The Uses of a Diagnosis: Doctors, Patients, and Neurasthenia," *Journal of the History of Medicine* 32, no. 1 (January 1977): 34.

15. George M. Beard, *A Practical Treatise on Nervous Exhaustion (Neurasthenia): Its Symptoms, Nature, Sequences, Treatment,* 2nd ed., rev. (New York: William Wood & Co., 1880), p. 85, as cited in Barbara Sicherman, "The Uses of a Diagnosis: Doctors, Patients, and Neuras-thenia," *Journal of the History of Medicine* 32, no. 1 (January 1977): 34.

16. George M. Beard, A.M.M.D., *American Nervousness: Its Causes and Consequences* (New York: G. P. Putnam's Sons, 1881), pp. 7–8. Beard lists some eighty symptoms along with the comment, "The above list is not supposed to be complete, but only representative and typical."

17. Gosling, *Before Freud,* p. 147. For biographical background on Beard and the practice of neurology in his time, I have drawn on Gosling, *Before Freud;* Michelle Stacey, *The Fasting Girl: A True Victorian Medical Mystery* (New York: Tarcher/Penguin, 2002); and Charles E. Rosenberg, *No Other Gods: On Science and American Social Thought* (Baltimore: The Johns Hopkins University Press, 1997).

18. Stacey, *The Fasting Girl,* p. 134.

19. Despite the fact that late-nineteenth-century medicine had a

distinctly somatic basis, that is, that legitimate disease was believed to reside in pathological changes in the body, doctors often listened to and counseled their patients, providing a bedside service in the psychological arts. Yet they focused on physical, not psychological, causes of illness. Reviewing medical records from the years 1880–1900 at Massachusetts General Hospital, for instance, Barbara Sicherman notes, "An occasional entry reported a recent death in the family but attributed the breakdown to excessive exposure to cold or rain at the funeral rather than to the psychological effects of the loss." Barbara Sicherman, "The Uses of a Diagnosis: Doctors, Patients, and Neurasthenia," *Journal of the History of Medicine* 32, no. 1 (January 1977): 52.

20. Stacey, *The Fasting Girl,* p. 142.

21. George M. Beard, "Neurasthenia or Nervous Exhaustion," *Boston Medical and Surgical Journal* 80 (1869): 217, as cited in Rosenberg, *No Other Gods,* p. 101.

22. Beard, *American Nervousness,* p. 96.

23. Ibid., p. 99.

24. Anson Rabinbach, *The Human Motor: Energy, Fatigue, and the Origins of Modernity* (Berkeley: University of California Press, 1992), p. 160.

25. A. Clark, "Some Observations Concerning What Is Called Neurasthenia," *British Medical Journal* 1886; ii: 853–855, as cited in Simon Wessely et al., *Chronic Fatigue and Its Syndromes* (New York: Oxford University Press, 1998), p. 106.

26. Interestingly, this is not the case in China and Japan, where mental illness is much more stigmatized than in the United States. In these countries, the term neurasthenia is still used and regarded as preferable to a diagnosis of mental illness. As cultural historian Tom Lutz points out, "The fact that neurasthenia is regarded as a protection against psychiatric diagnosis in some cultures and a dangerous slide into a psy-

chogenic diagnosis in others is the mark of its ability, as a diagnosis, to bridge this fundamental divide." Lutz, "Varieties of Medical Experience," p. 70.

27. George M. Beard, *American Nervousness,* pp. iv–v.

28. Ibid., p. xii.

29. Ibid., p. xi.

30. Gosling, *Before Freud,* p. 164, as quoted in Tom Lutz, "Varieties of Medical Experience," p. 74.

31. Lutz, "Varieties of Medical Experience," p. 74. In fact, attempts were made to subgroup neurasthenic patients according to cause and symptoms, but the results were unsatisfactory. See Gosling, *Before Freud,* p. 164.

32. Norma C. Ware, "Society, Mind and Body," in *Chronic Fatigue Syndrome: An Anthropological View,* Ciba Foundation Symposium 173 (Chichester, UK: Wiley, 1993), p. 81, comment by M. C. Sharpe. See also Norma C. Ware, Ph.D., and Arthur Kleinman, M.D., "Culture and Somatic Experience: The Social Course of Illness in Neurasthenia and Chronic Fatigue Syndrome," *Psychosomatic Medicine* 54, no. 5 (September/October 1992): 552, in which the authors comment on the way patients often construct a "biopsychosocial etiological model" when describing the onset of their illness.

33. Stacey, *The Fasting Girl,* p. 136.

CHAPTER EIGHT

1. A 1998 survey conducted by *The CFIDS Chronicle* rated the beneficial impact of interventions ranging from yoga to beta blockers to Klonopin. The top-rated treatment for people with CFIDS, effective for 98 percent of respondents, was pacing of activities, not doing more than you feel able to do on any given day. "1999 Chronicle Reader Survey," *The CFIDS Chronicle* 12 (4): 6. Second-most-helpful was change in out-

look, third was treating sleep problems, fourth avoiding chemicals, and fifth avoiding problem foods. Treatments with the highest percentage of "harmful" ratings were beta blockers, colonics, graded exercise, neurontin, florinef/midodrine, Klonopin, antidepressants, aggressive rest.

2. Robert Louis Stevenson, "An Apology for Idlers," in *The Art of the Personal Essay: An Anthology from the Classical Era to the Present,* ed. Phillip Lopate (New York: Random House, 1995), p. 222.

3. Kat Duff, *The Alchemy of Illness* (New York: Pantheon, 1993), p. 35.

CHAPTER NINE

1. Porter, *The Greatest Benefit to Mankind,* p. 309.

2. Ibid., p. 310.

3. Ibid., p. 311.

4. Ibid., p. 310.

5. Thomas Bodenheimer, M.D.; Kate Lorig, R.N., Dr. P. H.; Halsted Holman, M.D.; and Kevin Grumbach, M.D., "Patient Self-management of Chronic Disease in Primary Care," *JAMA: The Journal of the American Medical Association* 288, no. 19 (November 20, 2002): 2469–70.

6. Laurence Foss, *The End of Modern Medicine: Biomedical Science under a Microscope* (Albany: State University of New York Press, 2002), p. 4.

7. Sontag, *Illness as Metaphor and AIDS and Its Metaphors,* p. 71.

8. Ulrich Beck, *Ecological Enlightenment* (New Jersey: Humanities, 1995), p. 15., as quoted in Stephen R. Couch and Steve Kroll-Smith, "Environmental Movements and Expert Knowledge: Evidence for a New Populism," in *Illness and the Environment: A Reader in Contested Medicine,* ed. Steve Kroll-Smith, Phil Brown, and Valerie J. Gunter (New York: New York University Press, 2000), p. 401.

9. The field of medical humanities emerged in the late 1960s and

early '70s as an antidote to an increasingly impersonal, technological medical practice. In 1972 there were 11 medical schools with humanities programs. By 1980, 117 out of 125 accredited medical schools had such programs. These programs provide medical interns with training in the social sciences and literature in order to increase empathy, understanding of the patient's lived world, and the ability to weigh the practical and ethical impact of medical decisions. The intersection of literature and medicine has since the '80s spawned numerous professional conferences, publications, and organizations.

10. David B. Morris, *Illness and Culture in the Postmodern Age* (Berkeley: University of California Press, 1998), pp. 264–65.

11. Ibid., p. 264.

12. Melanie Thernstrom, "The Writing Cure: Can Understanding Narrative Make You a Better Doctor?" *The New York Times Magazine,* April 18, 2004, p. 44.

13. Kathryn Montgomery Hunter, *Doctors' Stories: The Narrative Structure of Medical Knowledge* (Princeton, N.J.: Princeton University Press, 1991), p. 159.

14. Rita Charon et al., "Literature and Medicine: Contributions to Clinical Practice," *Annals of Internal Medicine* 122, no. 8 (April 15, 1995): 599. While the authors call for further longitudinal research, the conclusion of their paper states that "Outcome studies of literature and medicine courses . . . have shown that such courses improve students' understanding of patients' experiences, enrich students' capacities for dealing with ethical problems, or deepen students' self-knowledge in clinically relevant ways."

15. While his young son watches, the doctor in "Indian Camp" performs a caesarean on an Indian woman, using a pen knife and fishing cord and without anesthetic; her cries are so horrendous, the treatment of her so cruel, her husband slits his throat rather than listen. The story raises complex ethical questions about treatments that degrade and bru-

talize the patient, about racism, sexism, and a doctor's arrogance and inhumanity.

16. Kleinman, *The Illness Narratives,* p. 114.

17. Jonathan A. Edlow, M.D., *Bull's Eye: Unraveling the Medical Mystery of Lyme Disease* (New Haven, Conn.: Yale University Press, 2003), p. 32. For Polly Murray's story I've drawn on Edlow's book.

18. Some scientists argue that Lyme disease was not entirely new, but closely related to a disease known in Europe since the early twentieth century, erythema chronicum migrans (ECM). See Edlow, *Bull's Eye,* pp. 55–61.

19. Arthur W. Frank, *The Wounded Storyteller: Body, Illness, and Ethics* (Chicago: University of Chicago Press, 1995), p. 25.

20. David B. Morris, *Illness and Culture,* p. 268. Morris cites Komesaroff as having used the term "microethics" and Cavell as being a crucial "guide to the philosophical implications of ordinary experience," *Illness and Culture,* pp. 268, 266.

21. Ibid., p. 268.

22. Ibid.

23. Ibid., p. 264.

24. Phone interview with Dr. Anthony Komaroff, May 10, 2004.

CHAPTER TEN

1. Kathy Charmaz, *Good Days, Bad Days: The Self in Chronic Illness and Time* (New Brunswick, N.J.: Rutgers University Press, 1991), p. 112. Charmaz presents a nuanced discussion of the complex issues raised by disclosing illness: the way disclosure affects self-concept, relationships, ideas about privacy, issues of control and acceptance.

2. Ibid., p. 33.

3. Reynolds Price, *A Whole New Life* (New York: Atheneum, 1994), p. 183.

4. Erving Goffman, *Stigma: Notes on the Management of Spoiled Identity* (New York: Simon and Schuster, 1963), pp. 4–5.

5. J. D. McClatchy, "Two Deaths, Two Lives," in *Loss within Loss: Artists in the Age of AIDS,* ed. Edmund White (Madison: University of Wisconsin Press, 2001), p. 225.

6. Edmund Wilson, *The Wound and the Bow: Seven Studies in Literature* (Athens: Ohio University Press, 1997), p. 223.

7. Sophocles, *Philoctetes,* trans. Judith Affleck, p. 21.

8. Wilson, *The Wound and the Bow,* p. 237.

9. Sophocles, *Philoctetes,* p. 35.

10. Of course, the stories of the Greeks are always streaked with wild contradictions. The same act of forgiveness that heals Philoctetes' ulcerated wound and restores order to the Greeks wreaks chaos and destruction on the Trojans. Philoctetes slays Paris and the Greeks sack Troy, an act of savagery complete with babies thrown from ramparts, wholesale slaughter, and the city flaming in a hellish inferno.

On another note, the backstory to Philoctetes' tale is also a story of alliance with the wounded. Heracles rewarded Philoctetes with his bow because Philoctetes agreed to light Heracles' funeral pyre, to release Heracles from the terrible suffering inflicted by a poisoned robe given him by his jealous wife. Philoctetes gained his godlike strength by an act of compassion, by overcoming his fear of someone else's unbearable wound, though here again, compassion and violence are inextricably entwined.

CHAPTER ELEVEN

1. Primo Levi, "Weightless," in *Twenty-One: The Best of Granta Magazine* (London: Granta Books, 2001), p. 158.

2. Ibid.

3. The Canadian 2003 clinical case definition for ME/CFS acknowl-

edges this variability: "Patients are expected to exhibit symptoms from within the symptom group as indicated, however a given patient will suffer from a cluster of symptoms often unique to him/her." Bruce M. Carruthers, M.D., et al., "Myalgic Encephalomyelitis/Chronic Fatigue Syndrome: Clinical Working Case Definition, Diagnostic and Treatment Protocols," *Journal of Chronic Fatigue Syndrome* 11, no. 1 (2003): 13.

4. For his description of the triad of CFS symptoms, see Dr. Paul Cheney's presentation "New Insights into the Pathophysiology and Treatment of CFS," sponsored by the CFS/FM support group of Dallas–Fort Worth and videotaped in Dallas, Texas, October 2001.

5. Joan Nestle, "When Tiredness Gives Way to Tiredness," in *Stricken: Voices from the Hidden Epidemic of Chronic Fatigue Syndrome*, ed. Peggy Munson (New York: The Haworth Press, 2000), pp. 41–42. Similarly, during the late 1960s and early '70s doctors repeatedly dismissed artist Polly Murray of Lyme, Connecticut, when she complained of swollen joints, rashes, and neurological symptoms, viewing her as a "thick-folder patient." "As her medical record grew thicker and thicker, doctors began to suspect that hypochondria was behind the aches and pains that came and went seemingly at will." Edlow, *Bull's Eye*, p. 3. Only when her physicians listened to her did they come to understand her illness as Lyme disease.

6. Anson Rabinbach, *The Human Motor: Energy, Fatigue, and the Origins of Modernity* (Berkeley: University of California Press, 1990), p. 160.

7. Norma Ware, "Suffering and the Social Construction of Illness: The Delegitimisation of Illness Experience in Chronic Fatigue Syndrome," *Medical Anthropology Quarterly* 6, no. 4 (1992): 347–61.

8. Johnson, *Osler's Web*, p. 197. For information on previous epidemics I have drawn on Johnson, *Osler's Web*, pp. 196–203, and Aronowitz, *Making Sense of Illness*, pp. 19–38.

9. David C. Poskanzer et al., "Epidemic Neuromyasthenia: An Out-

break in Punta Gorda, Florida," *New England Journal of Medicine* 257, no. 8 (August 22, 1957): 356, 363.

10. Ibid., pp. 357, 363.

11. Ibid., p. 363.

12. Ibid., p. 356–64.

13. Johnson, *Osler's Web,* p. 198.

14. Alexis Shelokov et al., "Epidemic Neuromyasthenia: An Outbreak of Poliomyelitislike Illness in Student Nurses," *New England Journal of Medicine* 257, no. 8 (August 22, 1957): 345–55.

15. Johnson, *Osler's Web,* p. 200.

16. Ibid.; A. G. Gilliam, *Epidemiological Study of an Epidemic Diagnosed as Poliomyelitis, Occurring among the Personnel of the Los Angeles County General Hospital during the Summer of 1934,* Public Health Bulletin 240 (Washington, D.C.: U.S. Treasury Department, Public Health Service, April 1938).

17. Aronowitz, *Making Sense of Illness,* p. 20.

18. Ibid., p. 22; Mary F. Bigler and J. M. Nielsen, "Poliomyelitis in Los Angeles in 1934," *Bulletin of the Los Angeles Neurological Society* 2 (1937): 48.

19. Hillary Johnson, *Osler's Web,* p. 200.

20. Aronowitz, *Making Sense of Illness,* p. 23.

21. Donald A. Henderson, M.D., and Alexis Shelokov, M.D., "Epidemic Neuromyasthenia—Clinical Syndrome?" *New England Journal of Medicine* 260, no. 15 (April 9, 1959): 758.

22. Johnson, *Osler's Web,* p. 201.

23. Personal communication from Dr. Anthony Komaroff, May 16, 2004.

24. Henderson and Shelokov, "Epidemic Neuromyasthenia—Clinical Syndrome?" p. 757.

25. Donald A. Henderson, M.D., and Alexis Shelokov, M.D., "Epidemic Neuromyasthenia—Clinical Syndrome? (Concluded)," *New*

England Journal of Medicine 260, no. 16 (April 16, 1959): 818.

26. Aronowitz, *Making Sense of Illness,* pp. 23–24.

27. Jonathan M. Samet, "A Conversation with D. A. Henderson," *Epidemiology* 16, no. 2 (March 2005): 266–69.

28. Phone interview with Dr. Anthony Komaroff, May 10, 2004.

29. Phone interview with Dr. David Bell, March 28, 2005.

30. Ibid.

31. Phone interview with Dr. Carol Jessop, March 30, 2005.

32. Phone interview with Dr. Anthony Komaroff, May 10, 2004.

33. Jason, "A Community-Based Study of Chronic Fatigue Syndrome."

34. Personal communication from Dr. Anthony Komaroff, May 16, 2004. He elaborates: "It was not until the 1980s that many virologists agreed that chronic infection that waxed and waned was typical of the herpesviruses—such as herpes simplex and the varicella-zoster virus that causes shingles. Prior to that time, recurrent attacks of oral or genital herpes were considered by many to be recurrent new infections with herpes simplex, rather than resurgences of a long-standing and latent infection. . . . The realization that the virus that causes chicken pox in youth remained silent in the body for decades, then erupted to cause an entirely different type of illness (zoster or shingles), was not really proven until the 1980s, and was a big surprise to many."

35. Dr. Komaroff points out, "When all the employees of an institution—the hospital in Los Angeles, the hospital in London—report in sick it's hard to miss that. But when that same number of employees is reporting to one hundred different employers, then we don't have systems in place to notice that. I believe that in fact epidemics of this illness have been much more common than they were reported to be in the medical literature. But they were not recognized as such." Phone interview with Dr. Anthony Komaroff, May 10, 2004. Dr. Komaroff's observation highlights the tremendous importance of sound epidemiological

investigation, which can't happen if an illness isn't taken seriously.

36. Phone interview with Dr. Carol Jessop, March 30, 2005.

37. David A. Shaywitz, M.D., and Dennis A. Ausiello, M.D., "The Demise of Reflective Doctoring," *The New York Times*, May 9, 2000.

38. Phone interview with Dr. David Bell, March 28, 2005.

39. Carruthers, "Myalgic Encephalomyelitis/Chronic Fatigue Syndrome," p.10.

40. Leonard A. Jason, Ph.D., et al., "Comparing the Fukuda et al. Criteria and the Canadian Case Definition for Chronic Fatigue Syndrome," *Journal of Chronic Fatigue Syndrome* 12, no. 1 (2004): 38.

CHAPTER TWELVE

1. Charmaz, *Good Days, Bad Days,* p. 91. Charmaz's book illuminates the way illness alters the sense of current time—depending on whether illness is experienced as interruption, intrusion, or immersion—the sense of future, the relationship to the past, and one's self-concept.

2. Dr. Paul Cheney talks about two CFIDS patients who went into a coma due to accidents unrelated to their illness and experienced a remarkable healing of their CFIDS symptoms. See "New Insights into the Pathophysiology and Treatment of CFS," a presentation by Dr. Paul Cheney sponsored by the CFS/FM support group of Dallas–Fort Worth and videotaped in Dallas, Texas, October 2001.

3. Johnson, *Osler's Web,* p. 112.

4. Ibid., p. 131.

5. Oliver Sacks, *The Man Who Mistook His Wife for a Hat and Other Clinical Tales* (New York: Harper & Row, 1985), p. 11.

6. Johnson, *Osler's Web,* p. 249.

7. Sacks, *The Man Who Mistook His Wife for a Hat,* p. 129.

8. Antonio Damasio, *The Feeling of What Happens: Body and*

Emotion in the Making of Consciousness (New York: Harcourt Brace & Company, 1999), p. 144.

9. Sacks, *The Man Who Mistook His Wife for a Hat,* p. 125.

10. Anthony L. Komaroff, M.D., "The Biology of Chronic Fatigue Syndrome," *American Journal of Medicine* 108, no. 2 (February 2000): 169–71.

11. John DeLuca, Ph.D., "Neurocognitive Impairment in CFS," *The CFS Research Review* 1, no. 3 (Summer 2000): 1. For my overview of the science on CFS in this chapter, I have utilized, among other sources, *The CFS Research Review* and *The CFIDS Chronicle* as guides to the relevant medical and scientific literature.

12. Buchwald, "A Chronic Illness Characterized by Fatigue, Neurologic and Immunologic Disorders, and Active Human Herpesvirus Type-6 Infection"; B. H. Natelson et al., "A Controlled Study of Brain Magnetic Resonance Imaging in Patients with the Chronic Fatigue Syndrome," *Journal of the Neurological Sciences* 120, no. 2 (1993): 213–17; G. Lange et al., "Brain MRI Abnormalities Exist in a Subset of Patients with Chronic Fatigue Syndrome," *Journal of the Neurological Sciences* 171, no. 1 (December 1, 1999): 3–7, as cited in Laurence A. Bradley, Ph.D., "Brain Abnormalities and CFS Pain," *The CFS Research Review* 3, no. 3 (Summer 2002): 3.

13. D. B. Cook et al., "Relationship of Brain MRI Abnormalities and Physical Functional Status in Chronic Fatigue Syndrome," *International Journal of Neuroscience* 107, nos. 1–2 (March 2001): 1–6.

14. M. Ichise et al., "Assessment of Regional Cerebral Perfusion by 99Tcm-HMPAO SPECT in Chronic Fatigue Syndrome," *Nuclear Medicine Communications* 13, no. 10 (1992): 767–72; D. C. Costa et al., "Brainstem Perfusion Is Impaired in Chronic Fatigue Syndrome," *Quarterly Journal of Medicine* 88, no. 11 (November 1995): 767–73, as cited in John DeLuca, Ph.D., "Neurocognitive Impairment in CFS," *The CFS Research Review* 1, no. 3 (Summer 2000): 2.

15. B. Fischler et al., "Comparison of 99m Tc HMPAD SPECT Scan between Chronic Fatigue Syndrome, Major Depression and Healthy Controls: An Exploratory Study of Clinical Correlates of Regional Cerebral Blood Flow," *Neuropsychobiology* 34, no. 4 (1996): 175–83.

16. "Research News," *The CFIDS Chronicle* 14, no. 4 (Fall 2001): 12.

17. *The Chronic Fatigue Syndrome Radio Show,* July 19, 1998, Roger G. Mazlen, M.D., host, with Dr. Michael Goldberg, WEVD, New York City, 1050 AM.

18. *The Chronic Fatigue Syndrome Radio Show,* April 25, 1999, Roger G. Mazlen, M.D., host, with Dr. Myra Preston and Kim Phillips, WEVD, New York City, 1050 AM.

19. Mark Giuliucci, "Neurotherapy: Rehabbing the CFIDS Brain," *The CFIDS Chronicle* 16, no. 1 (Winter 2003): 22.

20. E. Daly et al., "Neuropsychological Function in Patients with Chronic Fatigue Syndrome, Multiple Sclerosis and Depression," *Applied Neuropsychology* 8, no. 1 (2001): 12–22; S. K. Johnson et al., "Depression in Fatiguing Illness: Comparing Patients with Chronic Fatigue Syndrome, Multiple Sclerosis and Depression," *Journal of Affective Disorders* 39, no. 1 (June 20, 1996): 21–30. See "Research Briefs," *The CFS Research Review* 2, no. 4 (Fall 2001): 10; and DeLuca, "Neurocognitive Impairment in CFS," p. 3.

21. A. L. Landay, C. Jessop, E. T. Lennette, and J. A. Levy, "Chronic Fatigue Syndrome: Clinical Condition Associated with Immune Activation," *Lancet* 338, no. 8769 (1991): 707–12; M. Caligiuri, C. Murray, D. Buchwald, et al., "Phenotypic and Functional Deficiency of Natural Killer Cells in Patients with Chronic Fatigue Syndrome," *Journal of Immunology* 139, no. 10 (1987): 3306–13, as cited in Komaroff, "The Biology of Chronic Fatigue Syndrome," p. 169.

22. K. De Meirleir, C. Bisbal, I. Campine, et al., "A 37 kDa 2-5A Binding Protein as a Potential Biochemical Marker for Chronic Fatigue

Syndrome," *American Journal of Medicine* 108, no. 2 (2000): 99–105; R. J. Suhadolnik, N. L. Reichenbach, P. Hitzges, et al., "Upregulation of the 2-5A Synthetase/RNase L Antiviral Pathway Associated with Chronic Fatigue Syndrome," *Clinical Infectious Diseases* 18 (suppl. 1): S96–S104, as cited in Komaroff, "The Biology of Chronic Fatigue Syndrome," p. 169.

23. R. J. Suhadolnik, D. L. Peterson, K. O'Brien, et al., "Biochemical Evidence for a Novel Low Molecular Weight 2-5A-dependent RNase L in Chronic Fatigue Syndrome," *Journal of Interferon and Cytokine Research* 17, no. 7 (1997): 377–85, as cited in Komaroff, "The Biology of Chronic Fatigue Syndrome," p. 170.

24. Komaroff, "The Biology of Chronic Fatigue Syndrome," p. 170.

25. M. A. Demitrack, J. K. Dale, S. E. Straus, et al., "Evidence for Impaired Activation of the Hypothalamic-Pituitary-Adrenal Axis in Patients with Chronic Fatigue Syndrome," *Journal of Clinical Endocrinology and Metabolism* 73, no. 6 (1991): 1224–34, as cited in Komaroff, "The Biology of Chronic Fatigue Syndrome," p. 169.

26. P. C. Rowe, I. Bou-Holaigah, J. S. Kan, and H. Calkins, "Is Neurally Mediated Hypotension an Unrecognised Cause of Chronic Fatigue?" *Lancet* 345, no. 8950 (1995): 623–24; R. Freeman and A. L. Komaroff, "Does the Chronic Fatigue Syndrome Involve the Autonomic Nervous System?" *The American Journal of Medicine* 102, no. 4 (1997): 357–64, as cited in Vicki C. Walker, "Feeling Faint? What You Need to Know about Orthostatic Intolerance and CFIDS," *The CFIDS Chronicle* 13, no. 4 (Fall 2000): 1.

27. Phone interview with Dr. Anthony Komaroff, May 10, 2004.

28. These methodological problems are discussed from time to time in *The CFIDS Chronicle* and *The CFS Research Review*. See especially Nancy Klimas, M.D., "CFS Research: The Need for Better Standards," *The CFS Research Review* 3, no. 2 (Spring 2002): 5; and Kim Kenney,

"Believing in CFIDS: The Role of Research Methodology in Gaining Public Support," *The CFIDS Chronicle* 15, no. 2 (Spring 2002): 7.

CHAPTER THIRTEEN

1. Lynne Sharon Schwartz, *The Fatigue Artist* (New York: Simon and Schuster, 1995), p. 271.

2. Marc Barasch, *The Healing Path: A Soul Approach to Illness* (New York: Putnam's Sons, 1993), p. 57.

3. William Maxwell, "Nearing Ninety," in *The Best American Essays 1998*, ed. Cynthia Ozick (New York: Houghton Mifflin Company, 1998), p. 175.

CHAPTER FOURTEEN

1. The committee consisted of patient activists, researchers, and representatives from five health agencies: the NIH, CDC, FDA, Social Security Administration, and Health Resources and Services Administration. Since the early 1990s, the committee had existed as the Chronic Fatigue Syndrome Interagency Coordinating Committee (CFSICC), a more informal group. The charter signed to form the CFSCC instituted a more formal, and therefore more lasting, structure within DHHS.

2. "Criteria by Which a New Name for CFS Should Be Judged," submitted by K. Kimberly Kenney for consideration by DHHS CFS Coordinating Committee, April 22, 1999. Online document: http://www.cfids.org/advocacy/name-criteria.asp.

3. The attribution at the end of the online petition reads: "The A CALL FOR <http://www.petitiononline.com/mod_perl/petition.html> ACTION: THE RECOGNITION OF MYALGIC ENCEPHALO-MYELITIS AS A SERIOUS AND DEBILITATING DISEASE Petition to

United States Department of Health and Human Services, National Institutes of Health, and Centers for Disease Control was created by RESCIND, Inc., and National CFIDS Foundation, Inc. and written by Tom Hennessy."

4. From a flyer stapled into the center of *The National Forum* 3, no. 4 (Spring 2000), a publication of the National CFIDS Foundation. A disclaimer at the bottom of the flyer states, "The NCF is not involved [in this action] but many support it."

5. Abstracts of Papers Presented at the Bi-Annual Research Conference of the American Association for Chronic Fatigue Syndrome (AACFS), October 10–11, 1998, Cambridge, Massachusetts, Change the Name Session, p. 12.

6. Alain de Botton, *The Consolations of Philosophy* (New York: Pantheon, 2000), p. 186.

7. "Media Alert: 3/12/2002; Results of Recent Poll on the Name Change Work Group Proposal." Online document: http://www.cfids.org/advocacy/c-act_03122002.asp.

8. See their Web site: http://www.cfids-cab.org/MESA/index.html.

9. "CFS Advisory Committee Meets Again," *The CFIDS Chronicle* 17, no. 1 (Winter 2004): 11.

10. "Advocacy Alert: 12/11/2003; Name Change Statement." Online document: http://www.cfids.org/advocacy/c-act_12112003.asp.

11. "Message to Members," *The CFIDS Chronicle* 17, no. 3 (Summer 2004): 1.

12. My thinking in this paragraph has been stimulated by Aronowitz, *Making Sense of Illness,* especially his Introduction. See also Charles E. Rosenberg and Janet Golden, eds., *Framing Disease: Studies in Cultural History* (New Brunswick, N.J.: Rutgers University Press, 1992).

13. While some people insist evidence-based medicine will give patients more information, empowering them to make their own decisions and undercutting medical authority, with an illness like CFIDS, for

which evidence of organic pathology remains disputed, precisely the reverse is true. For people with CFIDS and other functional illnesses— fibromyalgia, multiple chemical sensitivity—a focus on physiological data works to encourage disbelief and dismissal.

CHAPTER FIFTEEN

1. Isaac Bashevis Singer, "The Washwoman," in *In My Father's Court* (New York: Fawcett Crest Books, 1966), p. 34.

2. Arthur Frank, *The Wounded Storyteller: Body, Ethics and Illness* (Chicago: University of Chicago Press, 1995), p. 77. Frank describes three narratives of illness: the restitution narrative, in which the body is restored to health, the chaos narrative, in which it seems illness and suffering will not be remedied, and the quest narrative, in which the person acknowledges illness, gives it voice, and finds in suffering a possibility for change and growth. Like others, Frank asserts that telling the truth about our bodies is a source of power, ethical action, and healing.

3. Lynne Sharon Schwartz, *The Fatigue Artist* (New York: Scribner, 1996), p. 9.

4. Kleinman, *The Illness Narratives*, p. 8.

5. Duff, *The Alchemy of Illness*, p. 57.

CHAPTER SIXTEEN

1. There is a vast literature on candidiasis, also called chronic candidiasis syndrome. See especially the writings of William G. Crook, M.D., and C. Orian Truss, M.D. I have drawn on their work and that of Stephen B. Edelson, M.D., as well as various online documents, for background on candidiasis.

2. The CDC Web site presents a glossary of terms most often

encountered in relation to CFS. Under "candida albicans" it says: "A common saprophyte of the digestive tract and female urogenital tract. It does not ordinarily cause disease, but may do so following a disruption of bacterial flora of the body, or in patients with depressed immune systems."

3. Phone interview with Dr. Carol Jessop, March 30, 2005.

4. Ibid.

5. Ibid.

6. W. G. Crook, *Tired, So Tired and the Yeast Connection* (Jackson, Tenn.: Professional Books, 2001), p. 39.

7. Precise figures are unavailable, but specialists in the field estimate that 2.4 percent of the adult population, or roughly 4.8 million, have fibromyalgia. The National Academy of Sciences has suggested some 15 to 20 percent of the adult population has some sensitivity to chemicals. If those who are made seriously ill by chemical exposure comprise only 0.5 percent of the adult population, that would be 1 million. Estimates of the number of vets with Gulf War syndrome range from 90,000 to 118,000. An estimated 800,000 people have CFIDS.

8. "Toxic Ignorance," Environmental Defense Fund, 1997, online report (http://www.environmentaldefense.org/documents/243_toxicignorance.pdf). In 1998, the EPA reported that of the 2,800 chemicals produced in volumes of 1 million pounds or more annually, 43 percent have no basic toxicity data at all; 93 percent do not have complete screening-level data. (Data provided by CALPIRG, San Francisco.)

9. Ulysses Torassa, "Odd Illness, Strange Clues: Autoimmune Woes Target Women," *San Francisco Chronicle*, February 18, 2001. Since the 1950s and '60s many diseases—such as Crohn's disease, multiple sclerosis, scleroderma, myasthenia gravis—that used to be classified separately have come to be seen as having an autoimmune component. This shift in view, as well as improved diagnostic abilities, has certainly con-

tributed to the increase in the number of immune diseases. Still, given the startling rise in immune disorders such as lupus, MS, allergies, or asthma, and a host of emerging or controversial illnesses linked to immune dysfunction—multiple chemical sensitivity, candida, fibromyalgia, Gulf War syndrome, chronic fatigue syndrome—it's hard to imagine that the phenomenal increase is due only to a shift in the way we classify or diagnose diseases.

10. Kenny Ausubel, "The Coming Age of Ecological Medicine," *Utne Reader,* May/June 2001, p. 56.

11. "Facts for the Chemical Industry," *Chemical and Engineering News,* June 25–30, 1994, as cited in Steve Kroll-Smith and H. Hugh Floyd, *Bodies in Protest: Environmental Illness and the Struggle over Medical Knowledge* (New York: New York University Press, 1997), p. 44.

12. Though there have been scattered efforts to correlate cancer incidence with hazardous exposures, there has been no systematic attempt to collect such data, even though the National Cancer Institute suggests that some cancer trends "may reflect changing exposures to carcinogens yet to be identified and clarified." Sandra Steingraber, "Time," in *Illness and the Environment: A Reader in Contested Medicine,* ed. Steve Kroll-Smith, Phil Brown, and Valerie J. Gunter, pp. 296–97.

13. Centers for Disease Control, "Second National Report on Human Exposure to Environmental Chemicals," online document (http://www.cdc.gov/exposurereport/introduction.htm), February 3, 2003.

14. Jane Kay, "The Face of Environmental Contamination," *San Francisco Chronicle,* February 1, 2003.

15. Ruth Rosen, "Polluted Bodies," *San Francisco Chronicle,* February 3, 2003.

16. The Collaborative on Health and the Environment, c/o Commonweal, P.O. Box 316, Bolinas, California 94924, http://www. cheforhealth.org/index.html.

CHAPTER SEVENTEEN

1. J. Joyce, M. Hotopf, and S. Wessely, "The Prognosis of Chronic Fatigue and Chronic Fatigue Syndrome: A Systematic Review," *Quarterly Journal of Medicine* 90, no. 3 (March 1997): 223–33, as cited in Renee R. Taylor et al., "Epidemiology," in *Handbook of Chronic Fatigue Syndrome,* ed. Leonard A. Jason, Patricia A. Fennell, and Renee R. Taylor (Hoboken, N.J.: John Wiley & Sons, 2003), p. 19.

2. N. F. Hill et al., "Natural History of Severe Chronic Fatigue Syndrome," *Archives of Physical Medicine and Rehabilitation* 80, no. 9 (September 1999): 1090–94. See "Research Briefs," *The CFS Research Review* 1, no. 1 (Winter 2000): 11.

3. J. F. Jones, R. Nisenbaum, E. R. Unger, M. Reyes, and W. C. Reeves, "A Population-Based Study of the Clinical Course of Chronic Fatigue Syndrome," *Health and Quality of Life Outcomes* 1, article 49 (2003), online document (http://www.hqlo.com/content/1/1/49).

4. R. Cairns and M. Hotopf, "A Systematic Review Describing the Prognosis of Chronic Fatigue Syndrome," *Occupational Medicine* 55, no. 1 (2005): 20–31, as cited in "Research News," *The CFIDS Chronicle* 18, no. 2 (Spring 2005): 5.

5. David S. Bell, M.D., FAAP, Karen Jordan, Ph.D., and Mary Robinson, M.S., "Thirteen-Year Follow-Up of Children and Adolescents with Chronic Fatigue Syndrome," *Pediatrics* 107, no. 5 (2001): 994–98, as cited in Mark Giuliucci, "Follow-Up Survey of Lyndonville Children," *The CFS Research Review* 2, no. 3 (Summer 2001): pp. 7–8.

6. See Dr. Paul Cheney's presentation "New Insights into the Pathophysiology and Treatment of CFS," sponsored by the CFS/FM support group of Dallas–Fort Worth and videotaped in Dallas, Texas, October 2001, in which Dr. Cheney speculates on the possible role of stem cells in facilitating the higher recovery rate among pediatric CFIDS patients.

7. F. Friedberg et al., "Symptom Patterns in Long-Duration Chronic Fatigue Syndrome," *Journal of Psychosomatic Research* 48, no. 1 (January 2000): 59–68; M. McKenzie et al., "Cognitive-Behavioral Coping Skills in Long-Term Chronic Fatigue Syndrome," *Journal of Chronic Fatigue Syndrome* 1 (1995): 59–67, as cited in Fred Friedberg, Ph.D., "Characteristics of Long-Duration CFS," *The CFS Research Review* 2, no. 4 (Fall 2001): 5–7.

CHAPTER EIGHTEEN

1. Andre Aciman, *False Papers: Essays on Exile and Memory* (New York: St. Martin's Press, 2001), p. 182.

2. Charmaz, *Good Days, Bad Days,* p. 138.

3. Frank, *The Wounded Storyteller,* p. 173.

EPILOGUE

1. Leonard A. Jason, Renee R. Taylor, and Judith A. Richman, "The Role of Science and Advocacy Regarding a Chronic Health Condition: The Case of Chronic Fatigue Syndrome," *The Social Psychology of Politics,* ed. Ottati et al. (New York: Plenum Publishers, 2002), p. 157.

2. Phone interview with Dr. Leonard Jason, September 9, 2003.

3. Presentation by Dr. William Reeves at the Seventh International Conference on Chronic Fatigue Syndrome, Fibromyalgia, and Other Related Illnesses, October 8–10, 2004, Madison, Wisconsin. As reported by Charles W. Lapp, M.D., "Research Section," *The CFS Research Review* 6, no. 1 (Winter 2005): 4–5. The figure on numbers of undiagnosed patients is also from Dr. Reeves's presentation.

4. A 2000 study of 120 general practitioners in the Netherlands revealed that only 10 percent of the practitioners felt knowledgeable enough about CFIDS to advise their patients. Judith B. Prins et al.,

"Doctor-Patient Relationship in Primary Care of Chronic Fatigue Syndrome: Perspectives of the Doctor and the Patient," *Journal of Chronic Fatigue Syndrome* 7 (4): 3–15. The study also found that "Only half of the GPs used the diagnosis CFS. The main reason for not diagnosing CFS was ignorance of the criteria. GPs reported self-diagnosis in 68% of the CFS patients. More than half of the GPs could sympathize less with the complaints of CFS patients compared with other patients. These GPs experienced more problems in communicating with CFS patients and judged co-operation and conduct as poor" (p. 3).

5. Renee Brehio, "Survey Reveals Physician Perceptions," *The CFIDS Chronicle* 14, no. 4 (Fall 2001): 11.

6. "Analysis of NIH-Funded Research on Chronic Fatigue Syndrome Shows a Trend of Decreased Support: Fiscal Years 1999–2003," document prepared by the CFIDS Association of America and presented to the Department of Health and Human Services Chronic Fatigue Syndrome Advisory Committee on September 27, 2004.

7. Personal communication from Kim Kenney McCleary, April 14, 2005.

Index

factors); produced by candida, 217, 219

treatment: need for, 247, 248, 256-57, 258; patient ratings of, 282-83n. 1

Truss, C. Orian, 296n. 1 (chapt. 16)

tuberculosis, 125

twin study, 71-72

U.S. case definitions. *See* case definition (CFS); Holmes 1988 case definition; Fukuda 1994 case definition

UBOs (unidentified bright objects), 2, 29, 173-74

undiagnosed patients, numbers of, 11, 69, 247, 256

vaccines, 226

Victorian neurologists. *See* neurology, in nineteenth century

viruses: and CFS, xvii, 23, 48-49, 66-72, 131-32, 175, 176, 245, 251, 275n. 2; and chronic aftermath, 71, 160-61; disrupting sense of self, 170-71. *See also* Epstein-Barr virus (EBV); herpesviruses; HHV-6 (human herpesvirus six); infection; mononucleosis

voice: of the body, 121, 248, 296n. 2 (chapt. 15); conflict over, xxvii; loss of, 37. *See also* language

Wallace, Marsha, 89

Ware, Norma, 154

"Washwoman, The" (Singer), 205

wastebasket diagnosis, and CFS, 9, 104

Western medicine, xxvii, 1, 9, 131, 162, 217-18, 248. *See also* medical technology; scientific medicine

Why People Don't Heal (Myss), 141

Wichita, Kansas, prevalence study, 10-11

Wilbur, Richard, 44

Wilson, Edmund, 141, 143

Wordsworth, William, 234, 235

Wounded Storyteller, The (Frank), 211, 296n. 2 (chapt. 15)

X-ray, 18-19, 118. *See also* imaging technology

yeast. *See* candida

"Yellow Wallpaper, The" (Gilman), 86

Yerington, Nevada, cluster outbreak in, 68

"yuppie flu," xviii, 246

About the Author

DOROTHY WALL is coauthor of *Finding Your Writer's Voice: A Guide to Creative Fiction* (St. Martin's Press). Her essays and poems have appeared in numerous magazines and anthologies including *Witness, Sonora Review, Bellevue Literary Review, Prairie Schooner, Cimarron Review,* and *Under the Sun.* She has taught poetry and fiction writing 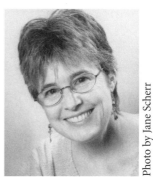 at San Francisco State University, U.C. Berkeley Extension, and Napa Valley College. She works as a writing consultant in Berkeley, California.

Photo by Jane Scherr

NANCY KLIMAS, M.D., is professor of medicine, psychology, microbiology, and immunology at the University of Miami School of Medicine, where she directed one of the Chronic Fatigue Syndrome Research Centers sponsored by the National Institutes of Health. She is collaborating with an international group of clinicians on a natural history study of CFS and continues to work in this country and abroad to bring a better understanding of CFS to clinicians and policy makers.